Diary
of a Midwife

To Rose
With best wishes,
Juliana von

Diary
of a Midwife

The Power of
Positive Childbearing

JULIANA VAN OLPHEN-FEHR

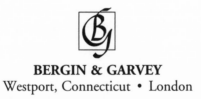

BERGIN & GARVEY
Westport, Connecticut • London

Library of Congress Cataloging-in-Publication Data

Van Olphen-Fehr, Juliana
    Diary of a midwife : the power of positive childbearing / Juliana
van Olphen-Fehr.
      p.   cm.
    Includes bibliographical references and index.
    ISBN 0–89789–588–6 (alk. paper)
    1. Van Olphen-Fehr, Juliana—Diaries.   2. Midwives—Virginia—
Diaries.   3. Midwives—Virginia—Biography.   4. Midwifery.
5. Obstetrics.   I. Title.
RG961.V8V36   1998
618.2'0233—dc21   98–3358
[B]

British Library Cataloguing in Publication Data is available.

Library of Congress Catalog Card Number: 98–3358
ISBN: 0–89789–588–6

First published in 1998

Bergin & Garvey, 88 Post Road West, Westport, CT 06881
An imprint of Greenwood Publishing Group, Inc.

Printed in the United States of America

The paper used in this book complies with the
Permanent Paper Standard issued by the National
Information Standards Organization (Z39.48–1984).

10 9 8 7 6 5 4 3 2 1

Note: Most of the names of individuals in this book have been changed.

With love and gratitude I dedicate this book to:

My Mother
Guliana Benjamina van Olphen Scharp

My Father
Hendrik van Olphen

and

My Husband
Eric Michael Fehr

The woman about to become a mother, or with her newborn infant upon her bosom, should be the object of trembling care and sympathy wherever she bears her tender burden or stretches her aching limbs. . . . God forbid that any member of the profession to which she trusts her life, doubly precious at that eventful period, should hazard it negligently, unadvisedly or selfishly.

Oliver Wendell Holmes

PREFACE

"YOU NEED TO write a preface to this book," my editor told me one early fall morning. "Tell us how things have changed."

I was in my office. A year before, I had left the beauty, sustenance, and excitement of my home birth practice. Now I have a computer and a white wall with diplomas on it. I go to meetings and I travel out of the range of my beeper. No longer do I hear the sounds, see the joy, or feel the awe of birth.

Why have I left the privileged position of helping another to be born? I could say that I wanted to leave the "covered wagon" of my practice for the swivel chair of my office. However, deep down I know that my evolution from home birth midwife to coordinator of the first nurse-midwifery graduate education program in my state reflects the power of mothers who have sent me forward to be their spokesperson and to guide the hands of new midwives.

Even though changes have taken place in health care that have enabled me to lead this educational program, not enough has changed to allow all women and babies to have the healthy birthing experience that is their right.

In the United States today, approximately 30 percent of women are estimated to receive inadequate prenatal care. Although our country has seen a decline in infant mortality between 1962 and 1994, its relative position in the ranking in infant mortality rates of developed countries with populations over 2.5 million residents has steadily worsened from twelfth in 1962 to twenty-first in 1994 (Gabay and Wolfe, 1997, p. 389).

What is the difference between the United States and the countries that perform better in terms of infant mortality? All of those countries have some form of a national health program, and midwives provide much of the prenatal and labor and delivery care in all except Canada (Gabay and Wolfe, 1997, p. 389). With 51 educational programs accredited by the American College of Nurse-Midwives (ACNM) in the United States that graduate over 400 nurse-midwives a year and scores of other educational programs that graduate other professional midwives every year, we have reason to believe that midwifery will prosper in our country as we enter the twenty-first century. Indeed, in the last five years, the number of births attended by certified nurse-midwives (CNMs) has increased by 15 percent (American College of Nurse-Midwives, September/October 1997, p. 1).

But we have to be cautious. The healthcare system in which we work is complicated. It is not a national system. It is based on the profit motive, therefore it shares the major concern of any big business: "the bottom line." Luckily, CNMs are the champions of cost-effective care. Although almost one quarter of women who deliver in the United States will have a cesarean section (Gabay and Wolfe, 1997, p. 389), the national cesarean section rate for nurse-midwife–assisted births is just 11.6 percent (Thompson, 1997, p. 12). The nurse-midwife vaginal birth after cesarean rate is 68.9 percent, whereas the national average is 24.9 percent (Thompson, 1997, p. 12). Also, our epidural rate is 14.6 percent and our episiotomy rate is 30.1 percent, both figures well below the national average (Thompson, 1997, p. 12). With these percentages, if CNMs were to care for even 25 percent of the population in the United States, the cost savings would be $300 million annually (Thompson, 1997, p. 13). If direct entry midwives (midwives who enter the profession directly from independent midwifery schools or through apprenticeship) are added to the equation, Americans would save $2.4 billion annually if only 20 percent of women increased their access to midwives (Blevins, 1995, p. 12).

Numerous studies show that nurse-midwifery care results in outcomes similar to those achieved by physicians while using fewer interventions and achieving greater patient satisfaction with care (Gabay and Wolfe, 1997, p. 393). In 1993, Butler, Abrams, Parker, Roberts, Parker and Laros published a study in the *American Journal of Obstetrics and Gynecology* comparing midwife-managed patients with physician-managed patients (Gabay and Wolfe, 1997, p. 390). These researchers found that within the study nurse-midwifery care resulted in 9.8 percent of the deliveries by cesarean section compared to 12.3 percent of those in the care of physicians (Gabay and Wolfe, 1997, p. 390). Even if the patients were compared by age, number of pregnancies, ethnicity and birth weight, those patients who were cared for by nurse-midwives were significantly less likely to have a cesarean section, less likely to have epidural anesthesia, and less likely to have an episiotomy and their babies were not at higher risk for a poorer outcome than those in the physician-managed group (Gabay and Wolfe, 1997, p. 390).

In 1996, Turnbull, Holmes, Shields, Cheyne, Twaddle and Gilmour published a study in *Lancet* in which 1,299 pregnant women who had no medical or obstetrical complications were randomly assigned to midwife-managed care or shared care between midwives and physicians (Gabay and Wolfe, 1997, p. 391). The authors concluded that the midwife-managed group had

similar or reduced rates of interventions, similar outcomes, similar complications for mother and baby and greater satisfaction with care when compared to the other group (Gabay and Wolfe, 1997, p. 391).

Another study that was published in the *American Journal of Public Health*
in 1992 studied the outcomes of 1,700 home births attended by direct-entry
midwives. At-home midwifery assisted births were found to be as safe as
physician-attended hospital births (Blevins, 1995, p. 12). Even when the
researchers excluded the physicians' high-risk cases and compared their low-
risk deliveries with those of the midwives, the midwives' home births were
as safe as the physician-attended births; but the physician-attended births
were 10 times more likely to require medical intervention (cesarean, forceps
and vacuum extractor deliveries) than those of the midwives (Blevins, 1995,
p. 12).

A study by the National Center for Health Statistics, authored by Marian
F. McDorman and Gopal K. Singh, released in the May 1998 issue of the
Journal of Epidemiology and Community Health suggests that nurse-midwifery
care may even be better than physician care. This study compared infant
mortality risks for all births attended by CNMs against births attended by
physicians. After accounting for a wide variety of social and medical risk
factors, the study of 3.9 million single, vaginal births of 35 to 43 weeks
gestation in 1991 found that those attended by CNMs showed a 19 percent
lower infant mortality rate, a 33 percent lower neonatal mortality rate, and
a 31 percent lower risk of delivering a low birthweight baby among nurse-
midwife deliveries than physician-attended deliveries (McDorman and Singh,
1998). The authors speculate that the differences in birth outcomes may be
explained in part by our prenatal, and labor and delivery care. Certified nurse-
midwives spend more time with their patients and remain at the side of the
women in labor while physicians' care is more episodic (McDorman and
Singh, 1998).

Now that managed care organizations are turning a curious, speculative
eye toward midwives, much work needs to be done. For example, even
though CNMs are legal practitioners in every state, we still have trouble
obtaining hospital privileges, prescriptive authority and mandated third party
reimbursement. Although many states have these privileges in place for
CNMs, most are controlled by physicians. We still face obstacles performing
births in any environment whether it is the hospital, a freestanding birth
center or the home. Usually, we cannot practice unless we have express physician approval in the form of signed protocols (plans of care), signatures of
approval for our prescriptive authority, physician cosignatures on our patient

care orders, or physician approval and support for obtaining and maintaining hospital privileges.

It has been argued that midwives need physician supervision to ensure quality care. But the research has shown that midwives provide quality care, and our national organizations have quality control mechanisms to ensure our continued competence such as accreditation of education programs, certification exams, continuing education programs and standards of practice. With these safeguards in place, physician supervision of midwives is as unnecessary as well-qualified drivers needing to drive with learners' permits. According to H. C. Lawrence, M.D., a co-chair of the American College of Obstetricians and Gynecologists Advisory Group on Collaborative Practice,

> By having the expertise to meet the evolving needs of women, each provider may assume responsibility for the care of his or her own subset of patients. . . . The collaborative practice team will always provide the expertise as needed and afford better coordination to maintain continuity. . . . The most effective systems are not one provider over another but collaborative teams of physicians and advance practice professionals combining their skills to maximize treatment and educational strategies that can improve the health of women. (Gabay and Wolfe, 1997, p. 395)

If we want to truly reform our healthcare system we must end the government-imposed medical monopoly—the restrictive licensure laws that require physician approval, and regulation of our practice—that has prevented us from providing the full array of health care choices to our citizens (Blevins, 1995, p. 2). State laws and regulations must be reviewed and revised to ensure that some professionals cannot gain an unfair advantage over others in the all too important regulatory process. Our patients also must be encouraged to sit on these boards to have a voice about the quality of health care in their state.

Finally, the medical establishment argues that midwives provide unconventional care; therefore safety will be compromised. Our statistics precede us, our care is time honored, and the consumer has a right to choose her care. In 1990, 22 million Americans sought providers of unconventional care. Americans made more visits to providers who offered unconventional therapies than to all primary care physicians—425 million compared to 388 million visits (Blevins, 1995, p. 3). We see medical schools offering more courses in unconventional therapies and nonphysician providers of unconventional therapies are more visible, but we should be aware that medical schools rely heavily on federal funding, whereas training for nonphysician providers is funded largely by private and nonfederal money (Blevins, 1995, p. 3). Schools that offer training for nonphysician providers (such as midwives) must be able to compete on equal footing with medical schools for federal educational funding.

Even though there are approximately 4,500 CNMs practicing in the United States, more opportunities must be made available for the education of not only CNMs, but all professional midwives. Within these educational programs, midwives and physicians must be taught together, as described in the American College of Obstetricians and Gynecologists's Collaborative Practice Model, so that we all become accustomed to working together. We must all develop a joint mission to improve access to all forms of quality, cost-effective care.

Now midwives need women to protect us in our labors. Women must continue to demand the right to choose. My optimism for the future of nurse-midwifery in this country comes from watching midwives practice their art of being with women and listening to them and honoring the unique knowledge that each woman brings to her own care.

References

American College of Nurse-Midwives (1997). *Quickening,* 28(5) September, October.

Blevins, S. A. (1995). "The medical monopoly: Protecting consumers or limiting competition?" *Policy Analysis, No. 246,* December 15. The Cato Institute, Washington, D.C.

Gabay, M. and Wolfe, S. (1997). "Nurse-midwivery: The beneficial alternative." *Public Health Reports: Journal of the U.S. Public Health Service* 112(5).

McDorman, M. F. and Singh, G. K. (1998). Midwidery care, social and medical risk factors, and birth outcomes in the USA. *Journal of Epidemiology and Community Health,* 52(5), pp. 310–317.

Thompson, J. E. (1997). "Midwives: Listening to women." *The Nursing Spectrum,* 7(19).

ACKNOWLEDGMENTS

I WOULD LIKE to thank the following people who have made this book possible:

My loves, my life, my children:
 Anneke Carolina van Olphen Fehr
 Ahren Michael van Olphen Fehr
 Julian Hendrik van Olphen Fehr

My sisters, Carolina van Olphen Carpenter and Wilhelmina van Olphen Smith for knowing that what I was doing was right.

Michele Niemeier for her support and friendship during all of those years.

Dallas Cooley, Warren Johnson, and Vettivelu Maheswaran for always being there when I called.

Norma Sides and Anne Holliday for talking me through those long nights.

Jacki Rooke for walking down this path with me.

L. Zan Ruby for her wisdom, love, and undying patience.

Alvin Glatkowski and Jan Kirby for their moral support.

Donna Evans for keeping me straight on my numbers and my allies.

Stephen Ernst for his determination and guidance.

and

Brian Emstovsky for his faith in me.

Finally, I thank all of the women who gave me the privilege of being with them as they brought forth the lives of their children; and I thank their babies who gave me the happiness of welcoming them into our world.

1

"PUSH, JULIANA . . . push hard!" Eric whispered urgently in my ear.

He was holding me up on the delivery table. The room was dark. Only a small light glowed in the corner. A nurse struggled to tie my wrists to the leather restraints on the delivery table.

"She won't be needing those," the physician's voice boomed.

The delivery room was hectic. The nurse who had been on duty through my entire labor was leaving and a new nurse was coming on.

I was oblivious. I had only the urge to push my child out. The green wall tiles shone with the reflection of a single light. The darkened room was part of our plan for a "Leboyer birth," a gentle birth based on the philosophy of Dr. Frederick Leboyer, a French obstetrician, who believed that babies should be greeted at birth by the soft glow of semi-darkness that they were used to in the womb.

Hysteria welled up in my throat. My earlier fears gave way to a physical determination, an all-encompassing force that was more powerful than my mind. All I could do was follow the urge that came from deep inside of me and in doing so, I created an inner tempest. I felt powerless, yet at the same moment I held the strongest power known in life . . . the power to give birth.

I gasped for breath whenever my body allowed me. The physician in his scrubs was a dim bluish image at my feet. All expression was lost behind his mask. He was busy getting his instruments ready, preparing to cut the episiotomy. (Later I would learn this was an unnecessary surgical procedure designed to enlarge the vaginal opening toward the anus. I'm thankful I didn't know that at the time.)

I felt a sting at my perineum as he injected the anesthetic into the area he was about to cut.

"Feels just like a bee sting," the physician assured me. Easy for him to say. I heard the scissors snip. Eric grimaced as he watched.

The head was born! I looked down to see my baby turn to face the left before she came out of me. Her little forehead wrinkled and the rest of her body slid out.

"Oh, look Juliana, it's a girl!" Eric exclaimed.

The physician placed her wet slippery body on my belly. She almost slid off. I held her to my chest.

I felt numb and exhausted.

We had a "Leboyer bath" ready. According to Dr. Leboyer, a gentle birth also included holding the newborn suspended in a tub of warm water to simulate the mother's amniotic fluid in which the baby had lived in the womb.

Eric bathed her in the warm water and cooed to her gently. She answered him with short muted cries. The room was quiet except for their "conversation."

I laid back on the table and watched them.

"What's her name?" the physician asked me quietly.

I stared up at the stark white ceiling, "Anneke . . . Anneke Carolina," I answered.

They took Anneke to the nursery before they wheeled me out to the recovery room. They parked my stretcher by the nurse's desk. Eric had changed out of his hospital gown into his street clothes. He was putting on his shoes standing next to my stretcher, grinning his loveable, unforgettable ear-to-ear grin.

The physician barked out rules to us. Anneke and I were his first "rooming-in" patients and he wanted to make sure everything would go smoothly. We were going to be allowed to stay together all day even though she would have to stay in the nursery at night. Eric nodded his head but his face told me he was too high to listen. I felt empty.

Suddenly the physician stood up and turned to Eric.

"You'll have to go now," he announced matter-of-factly.

I struggled to raise up on my elbow. "Can't he stay with me in recovery?"

"No," the nurse interjected. "It's not visiting hours. You're only allowed to visit your wife during visiting hours," she instructed Eric over her shoulder while she was straightening my sheet. "And, since the baby is going to be in the room, you'll have to wear a hospital gown and cap to guard against germs. We'll show you where to get them when you come back."

I felt panic as I realized he was leaving me. He had to drive all the way back home alone, and we had just become a family!

Suddenly my panic gave way to exhaustion. I couldn't think anymore. I sadly kissed him good-bye and sank back onto the stretcher turning to stare at the green tiles until I was wheeled to my room.

Alone in my room, the silence was stifling. Anneke was in the nursery, Eric was driving home and I was here in a strange bed.

I got up to go to the bathroom, the anesthesia was wearing off and my perineum was sore where the physician had cut. I struggled to maneuver myself so I wouldn't injure it any further. Looking at myself in the mirror, I was surprised to see that my new status as a mother hadn't changed my face at all. My hands were sticky. I looked down and saw the blood of my daughter's birth on my hands.

I don't know how many hours later I heard the baby isolette being wheeled down the hall. At last my daughter was coming! The nurse gave her to me and left the room. I felt surprisingly confident. I put her to my breast and she suckled quietly and peacefully. As I watched her, my mind flashed twenty years ahead wondering what she would look like. I closed my eyes and laid back my head. I missed Eric.

Three days went by. Eric visited us in our hospital room but he had to scrub his hands with strong bactericidal solution and then don a hospital gown and hat. He looked like an alien. In fact, I felt sort of alienated from him. I felt intimidated. Our surroundings were foreign and we constantly seemed to be doing something wrong. If we lay on my bed together, the nurse would come in and reprimand us. I wasn't allowed to put Anneke on my chest to sleep. The nurses were upset with us for breaking so many rules. In short, my family was disruptive to the system and the system was disruptive to our family. I couldn't wait to go home.

But, when the time came, it felt strange to leave the hospital. After three days of being a patient and having the nurses control the times I could feed my baby and have her with me, I felt like she belonged more to them than to me. I hoped that I could do as good a job as they had done. When the nurse put her in my lap on the wheelchair, a wave of inadequacy washed over me.

The long drive to my parents' house in Reston, Virginia was fun and helped to dispel some of my worries. It was a beautiful sunny day and Anneke looked so tiny in her car seat. The seat belts hung loosely around her body and we couldn't get them any tighter. Eric and I sang songs all the way home. I particularly remember singing "Sunny Day" by Paul Simon.

It felt good to be going to my parents' home. It was a very secure place for me. However, I knew they would be moving soon, because my father wanted to return to Holland for his retirement. They would be leaving within the year.

My parents immigrated from Holland to Houston, Texas a year before I was born. I was thirteen when we moved to Reston. My father, a chemist, started a job with the National Academy of Sciences. My parents were excited about moving to Reston. It was a new "planned community" where the architecture was unique and the neighbors worked together in associations to maintain communal property. But over the years, this system went awry and neighbors battled constantly over the fate of their shared land. I really think it was this and the upheavals of the 1960s that made my father disillusioned with America. He turned back to Holland for a sense of peace and belonging.

My mother was another pillar of strength in my life. Her undying devotion to me was truly phenomenal. She was a pharmacist in Holland before I was born. She was one of the few women of her time who had a career. But a tragedy caused her to drop her professional pursuits and devote herself entirely to mothering. My sister, the youngest of five children, died at the age of eight months after choking on a "tiddly winks" piece while my mother was at work and a babysitter was in charge. She never shared her grief with me, but I became the lucky recipient of a mother who truly wanted me and dedicated her life to me. It was only later that I realized why she never left me with a babysitter.

Because my family was Dutch, we were always different from our neighbors. Dutch was spoken at home and we practiced all the Dutch customs and observed the Dutch holidays. And we socialized with my father's Dutch colleagues and their families. So, even though we lived in the heart of Texas, we were really never "Texans." We were always outsiders. Now, even as an adult, wherever I go I still feel that way.

Eric moved to Reston with his family when he was sixteen. He wasn't in my peer group, but because there were so few teenagers then we were bound to brush shoulders. Initially, I scoffed at him, but as the years went by he gained my respect and finally, after I graduated from high school, when he asked me to go with him to college, I accepted. We've been together ever since.

Now we were bringing our first born to the home that we partied in, courted in, and were married in. My parents were away on a business trip (Anneke came two weeks early and caught us all by surprise). When they arrived two days later, my father, who normally shows very little emotion, made quite a spectacle of himself. He hurried up the two flights of stairs to my bedroom, his heavy shoes beating expectantly on the wooden steps. He rushed into the room, quickly sat on the bed, and miscalculating his movements, landed on the floor. A moment of chaos flashed by. Was he hurt? He brushed away my helping hand and quickly picked up Anneke.

"Ah yes, another miracle," he said.

He brought her to the window so the sunlight would uncover all of her features. He held her up like a work of art. He appraised her. She was indeed an artistic masterpiece and yet a scientific inquiry. I felt like he was checking my math homework. My mother peered over his shoulder. Each feature was scrutinized excitedly at first . . . every feature seemed to come from my side of the family! Then there was a long silence.

"These must be Fehr ears," he sighed. My mother reluctantly agreed. Oh well, that was quickly overlooked. Ninety percent was "van Olphen". She was returned to me with a grunt of approval. She was accepted into the family.

All mothers remember the births of their children. A memory, conscious or not, stays with them for the rest of their lives. I believe this memory affects their mothering and the way they lead their lives as women. Anneke's birth gave me a sense of power. I carried her and birthed her, fully conscious and aware of my control. I was aware that I held a phenomenal power within me. I came out of my birth experience feeling that if I could have a baby, I could take on the world. There was nothing that was more difficult, more trying, or more satisfying. I could handle all that came my way.

Unfortunately, most women don't come out of their birth experiences feeling the way I felt. The common and often unnecessary forceps and cesarean section give the mother one message: "You are inadequate." With the sweep of a hand or the breath of a word a physician can cause a mother a lifetime of feelings of failure.

Women go through life thinking they can't birth their babies without the help of surgeons and their machinery. I feel sad when I hear mothers say, "I tried to go natural but they said I couldn't do it," or, "I'd be afraid to do it without drugs."

I feel frustrated when I hear women say, "I (or my baby) would have died if it weren't for my doctor and the hospital!" It frustrates me because I know that in a great majority of cases, last minute catastrophes can be prevented. Women's fears cause them to demand the technology and they become captive consumers of an obstetric system that is virtually their only choice for care in America.

Unfortunately for women and their babies, the obstetric system in America is an expensive choice and is not affordable to an increasing number of women. According to the Health Insurance Association of America, in 1995, the average cost of having a hospital vaginal birth in America was $6,378, and a hospital cesarean birth was $10,638. Those figures only represent the medical costs. The loss of earnings from time lost at work isn't included.

The cost of the obstetric system creates many of the problems that it is designed to treat. Because some women can't afford it, they have to go without the prenatal care they need. Without prenatal care these women approach their deliveries in substandard health. They are twice as likely to have low birthweight babies, and they have more premature babies. The smaller the baby, the poorer its chances are of a healthy survival, and the lower the birthweight, the greater the chance that the newborn will need high technology care. Delivery time is too late for the mother to get healthy, become informed, or take control. Often, catastrophe is just waiting to happen.

Unfortunately, at this point, the only things that can save these women and their babies are the surgeons and their machines, the very thing they couldn't afford in the first place! Now, the cost to society becomes high. In 1985, the Southern Regional Task Force on Infant Mortality stated that about $16 billion was spent on maternity care. Almost $5 billion went to physicians and laboratories and over $11 billion went to hospitals. The numbers can only be higher now. It's hard for families to pay these bills, so maternity and newborn care has become the largest source of uncompensated care that must be absorbed by hospitals, taxpayers, and higher health insurance premiums. In short, we all pay for this expensive care that could have been prevented by adequate prenatal care had it been accessible to all women.

The ultimate sadness about the whole situation is that it is hard for mothers to bond with their sickly infants because of the separation inherent in neonatal intensive care units. The mother's feelings of failure over having an "inferior" baby are perpetuated and the vicious circle of abuse and neglect is begun. Not only do we all pay with dollars, but we all become the victims because the real losers are the mothers and babies. And they are ourselves.

With these thoughts, I write this book so that I can inform women about the obstetrics system. I want women to take control of their babies' births. I want them to choose alternatives to the system. What are the alternatives? Out-of-hospital births are perfectly feasible. I am a midwife because I believe that planned out-of-hospital births should be made more accessible for low-risk women to decrease unnecessary hospital costs.

More important than changing the site of birth is bringing back the midwife as the primary birth attendant. Midwifery is a profession whose time has come again. Certified nurse-midwives, the experts of normal birth, are nurses who have received special training in maternal and newborn care and normal obstetrics. Federal, state and local governments have called upon us to relieve the burden of the high infant mortality rates in our country. The United States Office of Technology Assessment stated in 1986 that

Certified nurse-midwives . . . affect access (as well as quality) by providing person-oriented services, such as communicating thoroughly with patients, counseling, promoting self-help, and attention to patients' emotional needs. CNMs interact with patients more than physicians do. . . . CNM patients obtain care relatively early in their pregnancies and continue to receive prenatal care relatively frequently. CNMs tend to increase the amount of prenatal care their patients receive.

My own experience as a mother as well as a nurse attending hospital births taught me that there is a need for change in our birthing system. I believe I can say it better than any government agency. And that is why I have written my story.

2

IT TOOK ME a full week to fall in love with Anneke. My feelings remained numb for quite a while because I often felt unsure of what I was doing. Learning simple skills like diaper changing, dressing and breastfeeding seemed overwhelming. I just didn't know whether I was picking her up right, how long she should be sleeping or what her crying meant. Looking back on that time, I feel fortunate that I had support from my mother and husband. Because Eric and I were teachers, Anneke's birth in the beginning of the summer gave us two months off before we had to work again. That was luxurious compared to the time afforded the average family.

Once I finally fell for her, Anneke swept up my whole being. Suddenly I recognized the mother's intuition I never knew I had. In a sense, this self-realization was a birth for me also. A whole new world opened up to me. I felt peaceful and euphoric.

That lasted a couple of days. Then my life changed. I woke up from an afternoon nap. Anneke was quietly sleeping on my chest. The house was quiet. It was a beautiful, sunny day and the birds were singing melodies outside my window, but I sensed a vague feeling of discomfort. Suddenly a feeling of heaviness washed over me and I felt suffocated. I didn't feel like moving. Tears sprang up out of nowhere. I was depressed.

The heaviness culminated in a thud. I knew exactly what it was. I had to go back to work in two months. I taught severely and multiple handicapped children and I was off only for the summer. But I couldn't leave Anneke to be cared for by someone else. No one could do my mothering as well as I could.

I put my arms around my little baby who slept on my chest, blissfully oblivious to the hurricane brewing inside of me. Perspiration formed between her body and mine. I began to reflect on the last year. I taught seven children in the basement of a very old school. Often we had no heat. My hands and feet were always so cold. Many of my students, already sickly, fought colds throughout the entire winter from the constant exposure. Their handicaps placed them at the bottom of the totem pole in the school administrations' eyes so we were virtually ignored. I was frustrated by the desperate situation my students were in.

Often, when I pretended to be working at my desk, I would watch one of my students. My mind would flash on her life. Was she happy? What did she think about? Indeed, did she really think? What was it like to have the physical sexuality of a teenager locked into the mind of a three-year-old?

As time went by, I saw more frustration in my students' eyes. Their behaviors changed as the year made them older. There was more incessant rocking, masturbation, hallucinating and self-abuse. They had no futures. They were going nowhere fast. The only place they could go from my classroom was the institution.

Their frustration began to rub off on me. I knew it was too late for me to change their lives. I felt helpless and helplessness for me is hell. By the end of the school year I was coming home in horrible moods and many of my nights were sleepless. I couldn't go on like this. Yet I couldn't leave them either. In a sense, I needed to stick by them. I needed to find something that would benefit me and also them. What could I do? Little did I know that it would be my pregnancy and Anneke's birth that would give me the answer.

Throughout my pregnancy my already inquisitive mind had been stimulated, so after work I poured over every book I could get my hands on. Through my reading I became increasingly aware of the importance of maternal health to the favorable outcome of the baby. Mothers who took care of themselves had healthier babies. As I meticulously watched my diet, I realized that the vast majority of the mothers of my students were poorly nourished. They were either overweight or underweight. They smoked, drank alcohol, soda and coffee. They ate junky fast foods.

I also read about the technological birthing practices used in this country: forceps, vacuum extractions, pain medications, cesarean sections and epidurals. All of these interventions are hallmarks of what medical professionals claimed to be necessary to ensure a safe and healthy delivery, yet I knew our infant mortality rates continued to make a miserable showing against other countries.

One article I read, "The Cultural Warping of Childbirth," by Doris Haire, changed my life. Ms. Haire argued that unnecessary medical interventions could not only disrupt the natural processes of birth but also could cause damage to both mother and baby. She gave the example of anesthesia. Not only can anesthesia block the baby's ability to take that vital step to breathing on his own at birth, but different forms of anesthesia interfere with the mother's ability to participate in her birth. She can become incapable of pushing her baby out at the end of labor and therefore the baby might be more likely to be subjected to other potentially harmful interventions like forceps delivery.

Suddenly, I started wondering about the misshapen head of one of the students in my class. Donna's mother had told me that she'd had a fractured skull at birth. She had been delivered by forceps. She was now thirteen and it had taken us the whole year to teach her how to count to three. And then there was Sean. He struggled along in a body made severely spastic by cerebral palsy. He had been premature and his mother had general anesthesia at birth. As she put it, "They just knocked me out." Could these be coincidences or did their brains suffer from a lack of oxygen brought on by intervention sometime during the delivery process? The more I read the more I became convinced that the way to really help these children was to prevent their handicaps from occurring in the first place.

Of course, I continued to visit my obstetrician for my prenatal visits. He was a nice man and I enjoyed visiting him but he wasn't too informative. And I could see how inadequate his care was. He literally zipped in and zipped out of the examining room. I wasn't taught what nutritious foods to eat nor how I could prepare for my delivery. As I started to get nervous about my own upcoming delivery, I imagined how frightened I would feel if I hadn't educated myself about pregnancy.

Luckily I had my childbirth education classes to attend. Eric and I started our Lamaze class when I was in my last three months of pregnancy. I'll never forget the wonderful Monday night drive over the mountain range to my instructor's cozy little home. We watched the mountain blossom with new spring growth. Our instructor was a robust woman, pregnant and due the same time as we were. As we sat in her living room she taught us so many things. She was going to have her baby at home and I was mesmerized with the ideas she presented to us.

Home birth was not a new concept to me. My mother had most of my brothers and sisters at home in Holland. She used to tell me stories about her births at home and my birth in a hospital right after they moved to America.

I would have liked to have my baby at home, but I didn't think too much about it because I didn't think the hospital option was that bad. I also didn't have much of a choice. There were no midwives available in our area (the closest midwife lived too far away, about two hours). I was left to my own devices: reading about childbirth and dreaming about what I could do to change things in my special education classroom.

Still, I read a lot about home births. I learned that most of the babies in the world were delivered at home by midwives. But in early twentieth century

America, with the beginning of obstetrics, the doctors effectively eliminated midwifery. In 1900, over 90 percent of the babies in our country were delivered by midwives. In 1976, that number was a mere 2 percent.

Many proponents of hospital birth said that the shift from home to hospital births caused an impressive reduction in infant and maternal mortality rates. While it is true that these rates indeed went down drastically during the same time that the shift occurred, their decline can better be tied to improved nutrition, sanitation, availability to antibiotics, lower birth rates and better prenatal care. The decline of these rates has never been tied to the place where the woman gives birth.

As I continued my reading I learned about midwifery. Today's nurse-midwife is quite an impressive professional. S/he is a registered nurse who goes on to get her/his training in nurse-midwifery—the management of women's health. The training can take the form of either a certificate in nurse-midwifery or a master's degree in addition to the certificate. I read that many schools such as Yale, Georgetown University, and Johns Hopkins offered master's degrees in nurse-midwifery.

After her/his training, and successfully completing a national certifying exam, the CNM can be licensed to practice in any of the fifty states. The CNM can perform well woman gynecology as well as manage pregnancies, labors and deliveries.

I loved reading about Mary Breckinridge, the first CNM in America, who started the Frontier Nursing Services (FNS) in Kentucky in the 1920s. She and her colleagues rode their horses through isolated mountain passages to deliver babies in the homes of rural families. Extreme poverty was the norm in this area with many children and adults chronically anemic from infestation with intestinal parasites. However, throughout the entire history of the FNS, their maternal and infant death rates were lower than in the rest of the United States, even though their rural population was at a higher than average risk. The statistics of the FNS were so impressive that in 1932 the Metropolitan Life Insurance Company estimated that if services like the FNS were adopted nationwide, the infant and maternal death rates would drop by 60,000 per year.

Many more studies showed that historically nurse-midwives are associated with lower maternal and infant mortality rates regardless of the population they served. Proponents of the midwifery profession argue that this is because nurse-midwives provide a different kind of care, a kind that is time intensive and educational so that women can have more control over their pregnancies and deliveries. Unfortunately, the medical profession is so powerful that, even with these impressive statistics, it wasn't until 1971 that nurse-midwives were officially recognized as primary birth attendants. Before that, Mary Breck-inridge and others like her operated outside of the mainstream, serving only the poor.

Even in 1976, when I was pregnant, I had no choice. There were no nurse-midwives or direct-entry midwives available in my area, so I had to go to an obstetrician and deliver the baby in the hospital. I assumed most American women were in the same boat.

Now as Anneke and I lay on my bed with the afternoon sun sinking in the sky, I realized that all of that reading was merely the catalyst to change my life. Suddenly, all of my questions had answers. I saw why so many babies were born with handicaps, and what I could do about it. If their mothers could be taught to eat well, take care of themselves and be active during deliveries, their babies would have less of a chance of ending up in special education classrooms like mine.

My hopes surged. I realized I could make a change by reaching these babies before they were born. I could help pregnant women manage their pregnancies, and support them during labor and delivery. In short, the idea to be a nurse-midwife was born in me. I couldn't contain my excitement. For a while I lay there and said the word "midwife" over and over to myself. The word was magical to me. It was right. It was me.

It's unbelievable how fast I formulated a plan. I was an experienced dreamer and in a pinch it was to my benefit. It all fell into place so easily. Now, to convince Eric.

My husband understands my romantic side and considers it his job to keep me realistic. Somehow, though, I knew in this he would agree with me. He was pretty miserable in his job as a special education teacher, having spent the year teaching fifteen emotionally disturbed, retarded teenagers in a fifteen by thirty foot "renovated" teacher's lounge. He was burned out and desperately wanted to move on. He wanted to get his master's degree in speech pathology, but he didn't know how to go about doing it. I carefully included his goals in my scheme.

I gently peeled Anneke from my chest and set her on the bed. Her forehead wrinkled just like it had when she was born. She settled into the sheets. I raced into the bathroom where Eric was taking a bath. Remembering my episiotomy, I sat gingerly on the toilet to outline to him our new plan. Now, years later, I can still see his face as I talked excitedly. As my words gushed out, Eric began to look like he was having a close encounter of the third kind.

My plan was in four parts. The first year I would continue working while Eric took courses part-time in speech pathology hopefully at the University of Virginia. During the day, he would stay home with Anneke. I would pump my breast milk and he could feed it to her while I was gone. He was attracted to the idea of staying with Anneke. His love for her consumed him and he already hated being away from her for any length of time. I thought it wonderful that he would be with her. Their time together would set the stage for a close father-daughter relationship.

The next year I would work part-time and stay home with Anneke while Eric went full-time to school for two years to get his master's degree. Because nursing school is a prerequisite for midwifery school, I would also take courses part-time to start that process. Luckily we had saved one of our incomes while I was pregnant so we could live on that savings plus my part-time job for these two years.

After Eric got his master's degree, I would go full-time to nursing school. Anneke would be three by then and starting Montessori school (my family were avid Montessorians so it was expected that I would send Anneke to Montessori school when she turned three). Eric would work in the public schools as a speech pathologist and I would go to nursing school while Anneke was in school.

I knew that since I already had my bachelor's degree in teaching, I wouldn't have to take all of the prerequisite courses for another bachelor's degree, therefore I calculated that it would take me approximately two years to get my bachelor's degree in nursing. When I finished that, I would work for a year in labor and delivery to get my required experience for midwifery school. After that, I would get my master's degree in nurse-midwifery. During this time, Eric would quit his job or cut back and work part-time to be available for Anneke. In the end, Eric would get his master's degree from the University of Virginia and I would be a certified nurse-midwife. It seemed so simple it had to be right.

Amazingly, Eric didn't resist much. He knew that neither of us was happy doing what we were doing and that it would only be a matter of time before we needed to make a change. He had been a captive audience to my developing philosophies. And, after living with me for so long, he often knew before I did what I was up to. It was a standing joke with him that I always picked the path of most resistance so when he heard this outrageous plan, he met my appeal with a matter-of-fact attitude that we would only be young once and that, if we were going to be crazy, now would be the time to do it. We could always fall back on our teaching degrees.

What a man Eric is! He is the energy and spirit of my life. On that sunny day, he entered the bathtub an employed man and left the bath to call the superintendent to resign his position as a teacher. Over the many years of our lives together, his faith in me has enabled him to take extraordinary risks to help me pursue my dreams. He has always been my backbone through the shaky path of change. It is his love, his constant support and his sense of humor that has enabled me to take on the grueling job of being a midwife. I thank him with the sincerest gratitude.

The first phase of our plan flew by almost flawlessly. I continued to teach while Eric stayed home with Anneke. While he went to classes on Wednesday at the University of Virginia, my mother came to watch Anneke.

My mother's devotion to me envelops my husband and child, and even though she had just been diagnosed with Parkinson's disease, she drove two hours one day a week to take care of Anneke. It was important to her to be with us as much as possible because she and my father would be moving to Holland at the end of the year.

Throughout that first year of work I proudly brought home six ounces of breast milk a day. With continued pumping in the evenings, I left ten ounces at home for Eric or my mother to feed Anneke. This was before people talked openly about working mothers expressing breastmilk for their babies, so this was easier said than done.

Because there wasn't a private place for me to express milk on the school grounds, and because teachers weren't allowed to leave the school grounds during school, I decided to talk to the principal. Before the school year started, I made an appointment to see him. I wish I had a picture of his face as it dawned on him what I was asking. I presented my plan clearly enough: I needed to go across the street every day to my co-teacher's apartment to pump the milk out of my breasts. I would then refrigerate the milk and bring it home for Eric to feed to our baby from a bottle.

Breastfeeding? Fathers staying home with babies while mothers worked? These concepts were not imaginable. With a face as red as a beet he pushed me out of his office, muttering that I must ask the superintendent of schools about these types of things.

I was surprised to learn that the superintendent of schools had to be involved in this seemingly simple issue, but I made an appointment with him anyway. He quickly gave me permission to leave the school grounds for fifteen minutes every day to do whatever I needed to do. He also made me promise that I wouldn't tell anyone what I was doing. I left his office calculating that I could pump each breast for seven minutes and keep within the fifteen minutes I was allotted. It never crossed my mind that I could probably take twenty minutes and no one would ever say anything.

Throughout the year, during my students' newly created "quiet time," I would slip across the playground to my "pumping station." Teachers supervising recess on the playground would turn their backs as I hurried by with my bag of supplies. Sometimes I would get one or two sly winks. When I arrived at the apartment, I'd pull out my pump (Eric called it my bicycle horn) and attach it to one breast. Then I'd reach under the pump and pump my other breast with my thumb and the side of the glass jar, balancing the pump on my arm. When the pump was full, I'd empty it into my clean French's mustard jar, reattach it and start again. After thirteen minutes of pumping both breasts, I'd have about five to six ounces, which I'd put in the refrigerator. After school I'd bring it home, add to it in the evening and start the following morning with a new mustard jar. Luckily, Anneke was a small baby and didn't seem to require much more than that, and at four months we started adding juices to her diet.

The school year went smoothly, but I had to admit that by my first mother's day I was starting to feel restless again. For the second phase of our plan to start, Eric had to get accepted on a full-time basis to the University of Virginia to get his master's degree. We called the chairman of the speech pathology department constantly throughout the spring so she wouldn't forget him when they went through the selection process. She was always positive toward Eric but she never gave him a direct answer. Finally, I could stand it no longer. With Eric's permission, I called her up and literally cajoled an answer out of her about whether Eric was going to be accepted. She finally conceded that she was 90 percent sure he would be accepted, but she couldn't commit yet.

That was all I needed to hear. I quit my job effective at the end of the school year, and the month of June was spent looking for a place to live in Charlottesville. We found a cute little basement apartment in a quiet suburb near campus and moved in on July 1. I got a part-time job working in a rehabilitation program for retarded adults, and at the end of the summer Eric was officially accepted into school.

By fall, I realized how hard it was for me to leave Anneke, even on a part-time basis, so I quit my job to stay home with her. I suspected that it had to do with my mother's experience of losing a child, but I never was comfortable with the thought of having someone else raise her while I worked. We have continued to alternate working and staying at home so that one of us would be with our children always. Luckily Eric grew more supportive of this through the years as he saw how our children flourished by being with us.

With no income, I vowed to live efficiently on our savings. We lasted a year on soybeans, vegetables and fresh-baked bread before I finally resorted to getting food stamps and Women, Infants and Children (WIC) checks for Anneke.

I'll never forget the humiliation I felt when I paid for my food with stamps. Whenever I went shopping I always got in the line that looked like I could get through without getting noticed by too many people. I felt guilty getting the food stamps, so I promised myself that some day I would pay back the state with volunteer work as a midwife.

Anneke flourished during those years. Anneke and I loved being together, baking bread, cleaning and washing diapers. I would dress her in pretty second-hand clothes and take her for walks or rides on the back of my bicycle. I put all of my energy and love into her. She was the light of my life. I knew what I wanted to be in life: a mom and a midwife. That was all. I was already a mom, but I wanted to be a midwife so badly that I dreamed of it constantly.

Eric's two years at the University of Virginia were hell. He was drained all of the time. He looked so strained and tired. His psoriasis flared up and he had constant back pain. I often felt helpless as I watched him leave in the morning. All I could do was make sure he ate well and help him type his papers. Finally, his graduation day came. He had won the battle and secured his degree. He was so happy that he looked like a rose, and I cried through the whole ceremony. He was the most handsome, radiant person in the entire class of 2,000 students.

Now phase three of our plan had begun. In the spring of 1979, I was accepted into the University of Virginia School of Nursing.

After Eric's graduation he took the summer off to stay home with Anneke while I started nursing school.

At last, I was on my way to becoming a midwife. I loved the lectures on pharmacology, anatomy and physiology, nutrition and health care administration. We spent hours in classes on the various fields of nursing like pediatrics, geriatrics, medical-surgical and maternity. We worked in clinicals in each of these fields (a clinical is where students practice and perfect their skills in on-the-job training). I spent most of my time in nursing school preparing for my maternity clinical. I had read enough. I couldn't wait to do some hands-on work.

Finally, the day came for my maternity clinical to start. It was exciting just to go onto the delivery floor and see it firsthand. Nine of us met for orientation. The instructor was a young woman, an obstetric nurse practitioner. The morning started out with the review of policy manuals and the introduction of procedures.

Then the instructor dropped the bombshell: Because some of the doctors had been complaining that there were too many student nurses rotating through labor and delivery, she wasn't going to rotate all of us through that section of the maternity clinical.

I still can't describe my feelings as I sat and listened to her explain her system of rotation. Each one of us would rotate through two out of the three sections: three students would go through labor and delivery and postpartum, three through labor and delivery and the newborn nursery, and three through postpartum and the newborn nursery. She had us draw straws. The three who picked the short straws would miss labor and delivery.

I sat there stupefied as her straws went around the room. I picked one . . . it was short! I felt a surge of anger inside that blinded me. Tears sprang into my eyes. I bit my lip and held them back. I didn't hear any of the words that were said in that room. I was vaguely aware of some complaints. I was numb with disbelief. I felt that if I moved one muscle, my temper would blow everyone in the room away. I finally mustered the strength to get up and walk out of the room.

I don't remember my trip home. I must have looked a fright as I stumbled into the house. Eric and Anneke were lying down on the bed reading a story. I let loose. I screamed, beat my pillows, cried and cursed. Anneke reached over to hold Eric for security. I couldn't believe it. Everything I had waited for seemed no closer. My instructor didn't want to bother the doctors.

I remember that Anneke sat with me while I cried and held me like I was the child and she the mom. Eric was calm. He had been through a few of these episodes with me before since I started nursing school, and he knew that I tended to rage about injustices in the health care system. But this was different—it was more personal. But Eric reasoned with me, drawing from some painful experiences he had in graduate school. I remember him pacing the floor while I watched him from Anneke's arms.

"You need to move on, Juliana," he said. "You need to make the best of the situation. You know that if you harass your instructor, she might grade you poorly in revenge. It's important to keep your grade point average up so you'll get into midwifery school. Remember, the competition is tough."

He held up his hand to stop my protests.

"I know what you're going to say about the system," he said. "But remember, anger makes you weak and when your weakness shows, there's always someone who takes advantage of you."

I knew he was right. I needed to keep quiet, show my dignified side and benefit from the experience I was getting.

"And," he stood squarely towering over me. "You can't keep coming home ranting and raving like this. You're scaring Anneke and it isn't good for her. You've got to find another outlet. You need to start writing a journal."

And so my book began.

3

THE SUMMER BEFORE my last year of nursing school, Eric and I decided
it was time to conceive another child. Anneke was four and we didn't want
to have our children too far apart. We toyed with the idea the whole summer.
I knew I wouldn't want to leave this new baby with a babysitter, so my
concern was how I would continue nursing school. On the other hand, because entrance to midwifery school was very competitive, maybe I wouldn't
get accepted for years. I couldn't have my children that far apart.
I learned early on that the struggle between family and career was a continuing one.

One peaceful autumn day Anneke and I were eating lunch.

Suddenly, Anneke said, "I want a sister!"

I was surprised by her outburst. I didn't even know she knew what a sister
was. Eric and I had been careful to talk of our plans for another child while
she wasn't around.

I said, "Why do you want a sister?"

"I don't know," she retorted, "I just want one real bad."

That night I told Eric what she said.

He laughed and said, "Well, that settles it!"

Our baby was conceived that night. A few weeks later I started feeling
nauseous. I knew I was pregnant. It worsened by the week. One morning, I
had my head on the table during breakfast to avoid that now familiar diz-
ziness. I wondered how I was going to make it through school that day.

Suddenly, Anneke said, "Mom, what's a sister?"

I looked at my little daughter in disbelief and laid my head back down.
That's what I get for letting my four-year-old participate in my family planning.

So I was pregnant during my last year of nursing school. My baby was
due on July 11, 1981. It was perfect timing. I would graduate in May and
have some time off before the birth. Eric would quit work the following
September and stay home while I worked in labor and delivery. We would
be able to live on paychecks until September at which time I would start
work. I would have almost two months off before going to work.

Obviously, I wanted to have our baby at home. Throughout the three years we had lived in Charlottesville, I had become involved in the local home birth movement. I attended meetings and we socialized with families who had, or were planning, home births.

Eric was supportive of my choice. He hated hospitals and to him birth was not a surgical event. He considered all of those scrub gowns and hats he had to wear in the hospital after Anneke's birth ridiculously unnecessary. He also had bad memories from our separation during that time. Her birth was the only time that we spent three consecutive nights away from each other. He shared my view that a family's beginning is not a good time to separate them.

I was looking forward to giving birth at home. Our apartment was bright and comfortable. Anneke would be able to be with us and we would not have to be separated from one another. That factor alone made my choice for home birth easier. Anneke was going to be five when our baby would be born. I talked to her a lot about birth and she watched many films and listened to many discussions about meeting with the midwife. She went to all of my prenatal visits with me and I showed her pictures of what the baby looked like each month.

But it wasn't only my concern about family separation that I thought about when I decided to have my baby at home. When I did my research for my papers in nursing school, I became convinced that, for the low-risk mother, birth at home was just as safe as hospital birth.

While I was in nursing school I attended some home births with Laurie, the local midwife, as a way of learning more about midwifery. Laurie was a CNM from New York. She was a pretty woman who had just moved to Charlottesville with her husband. She was so quiet and dainty that it was hard to imagine how she had the courage to move to a strange area and attend births amidst the tremendous adversity the local medical establishment created. Although she stopped practicing as a midwife because of family and political pressures, I continue to admire her courage as the pioneer in the area.

I liked the experience of home birth. The mothers walked around, ate, drank fluids and socialized with their families and intimate friends. Their children played around them just as if it were a normal day. The babies were born alert and active and their mothers could hold them and breastfeed them immediately. Mothers were never separated from their babies or their loved ones. I knew, when we walked away and left them peacefully slumbering in each other's arms, that this was the right way to have babies.

When I was four months pregnant, I found out that I was scheduled to take my nursing boards (exams to become a registered nurse) on July 8 and 9. Needless to say, I worried the entire third trimester. Would I make it to the boards? Because they were offered only twice a year, I'd have to wait until the following February if I missed them in July. That would be impossible. I had decided to apply to Georgetown University's midwifery program and I needed to work a year to get my labor and delivery experience.

Most importantly, I worried about where I might end up having my baby. The boards would be given in a city three hours away from my home. If I didn't have my baby before the boards, I worried that I might go into labor during the two days of testing. Because my labor with Anneke was quick, I probably wouldn't have time to get home. I had planned a home birth but not a hotel birth.

I graduated with Honors from the University of Virginia in May. George Bush was the commencement speaker. When I walked up to receive my diploma, Anneke walked beside me to a standing ovation. She had attended classes with me for two years, sitting quietly beside me, playing with her toys. She had handled nursing school quite well at the ripe old ages of three and four.

After graduation, I rested and studied daily for the boards. Assuming I could go, I knew my pregnancy would distract me, so I wanted to know the material well. As it turned out, Ahren Michael, my son, was born on July 6, 1991, at home.

I had contractions for many days before Ahren was born. Even though these were the painless contractions of pregnancy that some people call Braxton-Hicks contractions, some of them were strong enough for me to have to concentrate through them.

I spent these days preparing for my baby's birth. I kept my house clean and made sure there was plenty of room for my attendants and family in the bedroom. I kept Eric near me as much as I could. I needed his calm sturdiness.

We had a birthday party for Anneke on June 28. It was a big party because I thought it would distract me from my worries. I made a piñata and invited several children and their moms over. Two mothers were due to deliver at the same time I was. Both of them delivered the next day. I was depressed. I tried a lot of things to get labor to start. I took lots of hard walks and drank jasmine and raspberry leaf tea. The contractions continued, but labor wouldn't start.

By Sunday, July 5, I had lost all hope. This was the week of the boards. I scrubbed the kitchen floor. I polished it until it was spotless. I took all of my frustration out on that floor. I was on my hands and knees for at least an hour. When I finally finished, I couldn't get up. I was stuck on my hands and knees with my big belly hanging down. I cried for Eric to help me. He got me up and put me to bed. I was at an all-time low.

At 3:00 that morning I was awakened by a long, strong contraction. I rolled over and kissed Anneke as she slept next to me. Fifteen minutes later another contraction came. Then another. Hope surged up inside of me. Could this be it? A few more came. Then another. They were strong. I woke Eric up. We got up and cleaned the house a bit. The contractions were coming harder and they were a lot closer.

At 4:00 A.M. we called Laurie. I also called Mary, a photographer who wanted to take pictures of births to publish in a book she was putting together.

Mary came first and set up her equipment. My contractions were getting incredibly hard. I didn't remember them being quite this hard with my previous labor. I was starting to panic. They were painful. I felt my body flash hot and cold. I felt the perspiration pouring out of me. I was starting to become unaware of those around me. All I wanted to do was leave.

Laurie came at 4:40 A.M. By then, Mary and Eric had helped me onto my hands and knees. I was rocking and groaning. I couldn't believe how much pain I was in. I vomited a few times. Eric was holding my shoulders. I didn't want him to let me go. I needed him so much. He was holding me up as I felt myself slip away in a whirlwind of sensations. I was no longer cognizant. The voices in the room seemed to come from far away. The only thing familiar to me was Eric and I clung to him.

In fact I clung to his hair. Somewhere in the back of my mind, I knew I must have been hurting him by pulling on his hair so hard.

"I'm sorry I'm pulling on your hair," I cried.

"You can pull on my hands if you want," he answered.

"No, I want to pull on your hair!" I gasped.

My contractions weren't stopping. One was right on top of the other. Suddenly, I felt a warm spurt of water between my legs. I felt the same overwhelming urge to push as I had felt with Anneke. My body was moving fast. It was going to push this baby out with or without me. All I could do was follow.

"The baby's coming!" I cried.

I looked up to see Laurie standing next to me.

"You can go ahead and push, Juliana," she said.

Eric helped me to a semireclining position. My perineum was burning as it stretched around the baby's head. It felt like I was being branded by a cattle brander. Anneke was still sleeping next to me. I pushed Ahren's head out and felt tremendous relief.

I reached for Anneke.

"Wake up! The baby's coming out!" I told her.

She woke up and looked around. She was confused. She thought I was waking her up for breakfast. She saw Laurie and realized that the baby was being born. She threw her arms around my neck. At 5:47 A.M., Ahren Michael was born.

He cried softly. Laurie said that he was sucking on her fingers before he was all the way out. She put him on my chest and he nursed beautifully while all of us watched. I couldn't believe I had a boy! I couldn't believe this miracle had happened to me again! I felt privileged. He was the sweetest little boy I had ever seen. His little spirit glowed so purely as he looked up at me with big innocent eyes, blinking against the soft light. I fell in love. He was, and will always be, my joy.

I rested until the next afternoon. My family never left me. My baby slept on my chest the entire time. Then Eric packed us all up for the three-hour drive to Roanoke so I could take my boards. Ahren spent the second and third days of his life in a hotel while I took my boards on one of the hardest chairs I've ever sat on.

4

DURING MY SPRING SEMESTER in nursing school, I landed a job at a private community hospital in the labor and delivery department to fulfill my prerequisite for midwifery school.

The hospital had between three and four hundred beds, and it was located in a middle class neighborhood. The patients were mostly white. The maternity unit had about thirty beds in the postpartum section, four beds in the labor unit and two delivery rooms. One of the labor rooms had been converted to a "birthing room" where a mother could labor and deliver in the same bed instead of being moved to the delivery room while the birth of the baby was imminent.

While I was in nursing school, many of my instructors and fellow students told me that as soon as I started working in the hospital I would see how risky birth was and how important it was to have a baby in the hospital. With their warnings in mind, I was eager to see if I would change my mind.

One of the first births I observed during my orientation left me with a heavy, foreboding feeling. When I came on duty, a couple having their first baby was in a labor room. She was at the end of her labor and was pushing her baby out. We kept her in the labor room until we could see the head coming through. Then we transferred her to the delivery room. We shoved her heavy body onto the delivery table, tied her legs in the stirrups, draped her with sterile disposable drapes so that only her perineum showed through a small hole in the drapes.

The perineum was intact and bulging slightly with the impending birth of the baby. The perineum is perfectly designed for birth. It has the right amount of stretch to allow the baby to be born and the right amount of resistance to allow the birth to be slow and gentle. But to modern obstetrics, the perineum is considered an obstacle. So today it was a sterile surgical area that was soon to look like a bloody battlefield.

Dr. Williams walked in, his hands raised to keep them clean after his scrubbing. He joined the chorus of voices coming from the nurses encouraging the mother to push as hard as she could. After putting on his sterile gown and waiting for the nurse to tie it in the back, he sat on the stool so that he was eye level with the woman's perineum.

Continuing to encourage the mother to push hard, he filled his syringe with xylocaine to numb her perineum for the episiotomy. As the woman struggled to push her baby out while she was flat on her back, he injected the xylocaine. It made her perineum swell like a balloon. Then he started cutting. His scissors traveled about one inch down from her vagina and then he curved to the left another inch to bypass her rectum. Blood poured down the drapes into the bucket at his feet. I knew then why the nurses warned me to make sure the drapes ended in the bucket instead of around it.

"Push, push, push!" the voices continued to chant.

The baby literally fell out into Dr. Williams' hands. She was covered with blood from the perineum. The mother's arms reached down to hold her but the nurse told her to keep her hands away from the drapes covering her abdomen because they were part of the designated sterile area that couldn't be contaminated. After the baby was cleaned and the cord cut, he was shown quickly to the mother then whisked away to the nursery. Meanwhile, the mother had to lie on her back for another fifteen minutes so Dr. Williams could sew up the episiotomy. It would be another hour or so before she would be able to struggle to a sitting position for the first feeding.

The episiotomy is the most common operation in the United States today. It is a routine procedure in delivery rooms all across the country with the rates in some hospitals nearly 95 percent of all births. Yet no one has proved that it is necessary for a normal delivery. Many doctors admit that it is done for convenience's sake, because it is preferable to sew up a straight cut than a jagged tear. Also, it hurries delivery. Without the resistance of the perineum, the baby just shoots out. But, when it shoots out there can be more tearing in the rectum through the broken tissue that the episiotomy has created.

Yet, delivery could be so much better than this. The mother could be taught good nutrition during pregnancy so her perineal muscles will be healthy and will stretch better. She could be helped into an upright position so she wouldn't have to push so hard, and gravity would help her out. She could be encouraged to slow down her pushing during the birth so the perineum will have time to stretch. Her perineum could be supported with warm, wet compresses to make it more supple. All of these methods will encourage the integrity of her skin and muscle and at most, she will incur a small tear that would need only a few stitches. In many cases, the perineum survives intact.

But women all over America will continue to receive episiotomies, losing blood unnecessarily, which weakens them. In most cases, their perineums are sore for days and even weeks, which handicaps them when they have to take on the full-time job of mothering. Also, many women report that their sexual relationships are impaired from the pain and will go so far as to say they feel castrated.

After I witnessed a number of births in the hospital, I developed a theory that has stayed with me since: It doesn't matter *where* you deliver your baby. What matters is *who* is with you when you deliver.

Dr. Pima is one doctor I would never want in attendance if I were giving birth. I think of her when women tell me that they want a woman doctor because they are more gentle. The gender of the doctor is not the issue. It is the sensitivity and patience that counts.

I remember my first delivery with her. When I came on shift at 11:00 P.M., Dr. Pima had a woman in labor. The woman wasn't dilated completely, but Dr. Pima said she was tired and didn't want to hang around any longer. The woman was only eight centimeters dilated, but Dr. Pima decided that she wanted her to start pushing the baby out. (Nurses are taught to wait until the mother's cervix is ten centimeters dilated before encouraging her to start pushing. At eight centimeters, the cervix is not all the way open, so it can swell and become injured as the mother struggles to push the baby through it into the vagina.)

As we encouraged the woman to push, Dr. Pima had her fingers in the woman's vagina, stroking the cervix in an attempt to push it out of the way. The mother became hysterical because of the pain that this caused.

We moved to the delivery room. After we shoved the mother onto the delivery table and strapped her in her stirrups, Dr. Pima started stroking the woman's cervix again. Blood was dripping everywhere. I looked at the other nurse and could see she was struggling to hide her feelings behind a professional face.

Dr. Pima couldn't get the mother to stop screaming. She left the sterile field to get forceps from the supply cabinet. (The doctor is supposed to ask the nursing staff to retrieve implements. Once she has put on her gown to deliver, she is in a sterile field and should not move from her place because she risks contamination.) While Dr. Pima was preparing the forceps she was mumbling about how the baby was just about ready to come out so she may as well hurry it up. I could barely hear her over the woman's screaming. Dr. Pima injected some local anesthesia into the perineum, cut the episiotomy and applied the forceps to the baby's head way up inside the woman's vagina. She began tugging, pulling and turning the forceps. Sweat broke out over her brow.

I felt nauseous. I stayed by the woman's head, trying to comfort her, but her hysteria rendered her oblivious to her surroundings. I was stunned by what was happening.

Finally the baby's head came out. The forceps were taken off. Dr. Pima handed the baby to me. I took him over to the warmer to dry him off. He was pale and whimpering softly. I leaned close to him and tried to whisper some kind words in his ear, but the atmosphere was so frightening that I knew I couldn't convey comfort.

His mother's screams had died down to soft crying.

"Is he all right? Is he all right?" she pleaded.

"Yes," I answered. "He looks okay."

I tried to stop my voice from shaking. I wanted to sound reassuring, like I had heard other nurses and doctors sound.

I busied myself with cleaning and drying the baby. He finally started wailing and turning pink. I breathed a sigh of relief and wrapped him up in warm blankets. I covered up the lacerations that I found on his left cheek and arms so as not to alarm his mother. I put the baby on the mother's chest but she could barely see him because she was lying flat on her back while Dr. Pima sewed the episiotomy. The other nurse, obviously appalled at what just took place, quickly took the baby from my hands and took him to the nursery.

This baby was the first of many I would see who survived his birth in spite of, instead of because of, the doctor.

Dr. Pima had a habit of tearing cervixes open. She relied heavily on this technique in combination with fundal pressure. In this technique, the nurse stands on a stool next to the mother and pushes down with all her weight on the mother's abdomen to push the baby down into the vagina. (I did this only once. The woman fainted. I swore I'd never do it again.) When this combination didn't work, Dr. Pima used forceps delivery or cesarean section to get babies out. She had no tolerance for the rhythm of birth. She arrogantly thought that her time was more valuable than everyone else's and not even the birth of a child would stand in her way.

One night, labor and delivery was particularly slow so the other nurse and I were sitting quietly at the nurse's station gossiping and completing paperwork. The outpatient department called. They had admitted a patient in labor with twins. They wanted us to hurry with the stretcher because she looked like she was going to deliver any minute. She was a patient of Dr. Pima's so I called her at home. I secretly hoped that she wouldn't make it to delivery.

We wheeled the mother to the delivery room. She was breathing hard with the contractions. Her bag of waters had broken and the delivery of the first baby was imminent. We encouraged her to pant so as not to push the baby out too quickly as we readied her for delivery. We called the doctor on staff who was on call for all emergencies. That night it happened to be an obstetrician. By the time Dr. Farrar entered the room, we had the mother on her back and draped on the table.

He had just enough time to cut the episiotomy before the first baby was born. The little boy was born eight minutes after admission and his brother was born ten minutes later.

The mother was wonderful. She had been so controlled, and she was elated to see her first-born son. I showed him to her, not even pausing to take him to the warmer first.

The second baby was born minutes before Dr. Pima ran into the room. She was madder than a red hen when she saw that she missed the births. (She would have to pay the other doctor for the deliveries and, of course, she had been awakened in the middle of the night.)

Dr. Pima took all of her anger out on the mother.

"Why didn't you call me earlier?" she admonished the mother. "Now you made me come all the way in here for nothing!"

The mother apologized profusely. Dr. Pima used very little numbing medication to suture the episiotomy. And she poked the mother so roughly that this woman, who had so stoicly and powerfully delivered two good-sized healthy babies, was reduced to hysteria over the stitching.

To be fair, much of what I observed was the result of doctors being harried. Doctors had full surgery schedules and office hours and frequently deliveries just got in the way. Because of this they sometimes used high technology unnecessarily to rush births. And occasionally they were sloppy with their surgical techniques.

The use of cesarean sections is a prime example of this. I was amazed at how many c-sections were performed. At the time I was working in this hospital, statistics showed a phenomenal increase. Between 1970 and 1978, the cesarean birthrate in the United States jumped threefold, from a little over 5 percent to over 15 percent of all births. By 1980, it had reached 18 percent. The outcome for the babies delivered this way did not improve with the higher cesarean rates. This convinced me that many of the surgeries were unnecessary.

Once I saw Dr. Williams open the uterus and, while puncturing the bag of waters, he cut the baby's head. I was repulsed! What if the baby's head was turned differently? Would he have gotten her eye? The cut was one inch long and required stitches. Imagine, in the first hour of this child's life outside the womb, she had to go through getting stitches (without anesthesia) for a senseless birth injury. This was just downright sloppiness.

An interesting side note about this incident was that the pediatrician present made every attempt to play down the cut on the baby, as if trying to protect Dr. Williams. While consoling the mother, the pediatrician said, "Oh, it's nothing, don't you worry about it. It's good that Dr. Williams got the baby out in time because its malposition could have damaged it further!" (This was a scheduled, nonemergency cesarean.)

Dr. Voight was a new obstetrician in the area. He was a passive and friendly man, and he seemed open to requests that his mothers had for withholding interventions. I wanted to like him because his approach seemed like a breath of fresh air. But he did so many stupid things that I shuddered when his patients came in. I didn't like spending an evening with him.

During my orientation he scheduled one of his patients for a cesarean section. She had had a previous cesarean section, so she just made an appointment for this one on her scheduled due date. My job was to follow the scrub nurse around. (The scrub nurse gets supplies for people during the operation.)

I couldn't believe how fast the operation went. It was only minutes from the initial cut in the lower abdomen to the birth. Before I knew it, I witnessed the birth of a tiny girl. She was limp and continued to remain blue after the cord was cut. The pediatrician gave her oxygen. Her cries were so tiny. The room was quiet. Thankfully, the mother couldn't see from behind the drapes. Dr. Voight assured her that everything was alright.

Finally the baby started getting pink, and when the pediatrician finished his examination he quietly turned to Dr. Voight.

"When did you say this baby was due?" he asked.

"It's her due day today," Dr. Voight answered.

"This baby's not due. She's about five weeks early. She's too young to breathe on her own. I'll have to keep her on oxygen, and if she's not doing better in a few hours, we'll transfer her to the newborn intensive care unit. She's premature."

He threw down his stethoscope and walked out of the room.

So the due date was miscalculated. An unnecessary cesarean was performed and a premature baby was born.

I watched all too many cesareans. Whether a woman received a cesarean section seemed to depend a lot on chance. Dr. Horton had a patient whose baby was in severe distress. There was every indication that a cesarean should have been done. He had the operating team and the anesthesiologist present in the delivery room to start the operation at a moment's notice. We all listened tensely to the baby's heart rate as it slowed considerably while the mother pushed during the contractions. But Dr. Horton was in no hurry. We waited. Finally the mother delivered a healthy baby girl, vaginally. Had it been another doctor, or if Dr. Horton had been in a hurry, the birth would have been cesarean.

One cesarean was so incredible that I recorded each event. If I hadn't, it would have been unbelievable. Here's how it went:

By the time I arrived on my shift at 11:00 P.M., the mother had been in labor for twenty hours. Studying her charts I was able to piece together what had occurred:

The mother, a patient of Dr. Cox, had been admitted at 2:15 A.M. Her bag of waters broke at home. A vaginal exam indicated that she was only one centimeter dilated. (In the process, she unnecessarily was exposed to the risk of infection due to the, at this point, gratuitous vaginal exam.) The baby was lying in a posterior position, its back toward its mother's back rather than toward her abdomen. Because the mother was on her back, her labor was doomed to be long and painful. Had she been allowed to walk and turn over onto her hands and knees, she would have had the help of gravity, and the baby's back would have dropped toward her abdomen. The baby would then have been in the right position for a quicker, less painful delivery.

Between 9:15 A.M. and 12:10 P.M. the mother received two more unnecessary vaginal exams and was two centimeters dilated. Her doctor arrived and ordered she be given twenty-five milligrams of Vistaril, a potent pain reliever used for labor. I should mention here that the mother wanted a natural nonmedicated labor and delivery. She was a modern dancer and kept in super shape. Later I was told that Dr. Cox spent considerable time in her room, and the nurses suspected he talked her into the early pain medication.

By 6:00 P.M. the mother had progressed to seven centimeters and an intravenous (I.V.) line was inserted to make it possible to give her more drugs. Her entire labor had been spent on her back. At 6:45 P.M. an epidural was started with four cc's of Marcaine. (The epidural is a form of anesthesia in which a small tube is inserted in the epidural space of the spine and anesthetic is injected into the tube. If inserted correctly, the epidural will numb the woman's body from the waist down, rendering her helpless in the process, often unable to push her baby out. This lengthens labor and makes the possibility of forceps or cesarean far more likely.)

7:00 P.M.—Nine more cc's of Marcaine were added to the epidural. Because Marcaine is similar to novocaine, it lasts only a few hours and has to be injected periodically.

8:00 P.M.—The fetal monitor was inserted. (The internal fetal monitor is inserted into the baby's scalp through the mother's vagina.) The mother was still on her back. Occasionally we turned her onto her side. Because her body was numb from the waist down, she couldn't move on her own.

8:05 P.M.—The pitocin drip was started at three drips per minute. (Pitocin is a potent synthetic hormone which helps the uterus contract. Its use is a common consequence of epidurals. The uterus stops contracting effectively, so pitocin must be given to continue labor.) Pitocin can be hazardous because too much will cause the uterus to stay in a contracted state for too long, cutting off oxygen to the baby. For this reason a pitocin drip has to be monitored very closely.

Dr. Cox ordered the drip to be started because he felt the birth was progressing too slowly. The bag of waters was broken for over twelve hours, and the doctor wanted her delivered before the uterus got infected. (Even then, research was showing that too many vaginal exams during the birth could cause infections. Many studies were advising doctors to avoid vaginal exams and wait twenty-four hours after the waters break before stimulating labor.)

9:35 P.M.—The mother's cervix was seven to eight centimeters dilated. Her pitocin drip was increased to fourteen drops per minute.

10:05 P.M.—The mother was eight to nine centimeters dilated.

11:00 P.M.—I came on shift. The evening nurses told me that the mother had been okay until they had to leave her alone with Dr. Cox between 6:00 P.M. and 6:45 P.M. because they both had to be present for a twin delivery. When they came back, Dr. Cox had an epidural set up and had planted the seeds for a cesarean section in the mother's mind.

When I went to her room, she was still on her back and had been there since the internal fetal monitor had been applied at 9:00 P.M.

Dr. Cox's threats to perform a cesarean were rampant by now. He told her if there was no progress by 12:45 A.M., he would do the cesarean, and he wrote on her chart "NO ICE CHIPS ALLOWED!" He left to sleep in the doctor's lounge. By now it had been at least eighteen hours since she had anything to eat and she was left alone.

This mother needed support and encouragement. She needed someone to help her through this difficult labor. After all, this was her first time and no matter how much preparation has been done ahead of time, it's next to impossible to labor alone. Many people say to me, "But their husbands are with them! They aren't alone!" I answer that this is the husband's first time also. We can't expect him to take over the role of a midwife. Adequate support by trained people can prevent the need for pain medications that often handicap and disorient mothers, compromise their labors and necessitate the use of interventions that can harm both the mother and the baby.

12:30 A.M.—The mother's epidural was wearing off. She began screaming for Dr. Cox. Her husband sat next to her looking drained and helpless. He was scared. Everything had gone wrong from the beginning.

I left to find Dr. Cox. He was in the doctor's lounge watching TV.

"Your patient would like to have her epidural boosted," I told him.

"Tell her I'll be there in about a half an hour," he answered, not taking his eyes off the TV.

"She's pretty desperate. We can't seem to stop her from screaming," I told him.

He sighed as he got up from his chair, muttering about how women always seem to act like the epidural was cocaine. "Once you give it to them, they scream for more," he complained.

I felt like saying, "Well, if you feel that way about it, why are you pushing it?" Instead I quietly followed him to her room.

12:45 A.M.—Six cc's of Marcaine were added to the epidural. (Whenever Marcaine was added to the epidural, I had to take the woman's blood pressure every five minutes for forty minutes. This is done because the mother's blood pressure can become dangerously low when the medicine is injected into her spine. Also, the baby's heart rate can fall exceedingly low.)

The mother was now almost completely dilated. Only a rim of the cervix was left. Dr. Cox told her to push with contractions even though there was still a rim left. She was numb from the waist down so her ability to push was severely hampered.

Dr. Cox put his fingers in her vagina and tried to push back the rim of the cervix while she pushed.

1:45 A.M.—We moved the mother to the birthing chair in the delivery room. (A birthing chair is a mechanical chair that can be put in a variety of positions, including flat so that the woman is on her back with her legs strapped in the stirrups, just like a delivery table.) I was surprised by Cox's decision to move her to the birthing chair. She certainly wasn't a candidate for delivering in it with her inability to sit up and all of those wires from the internal monitor coming out of her vagina. In fact, within minutes of moving her to the birthing chair, we had to place it in the delivery table position.

When we moved her, the screw of the internal fetal monitor loosened in the baby's scalp so I had to monitor the baby myself every five minutes. I also had to take the mother's blood pressure every fifteen minutes and mark every contraction on the monitor because the machine wasn't working right.

Dr. Cox was still muttering about a cesarean, but he decided she could labor for a little while longer. We set up for a vacuum extraction. (In a delivery by vacuum extraction, a suction cup that looks like a plumber's helper is applied to the baby's scalp and the baby is pulled out of the mother. It is used in place of forceps, but it is almost impossible to turn a baby to face the right position with it.

Dr. Cox warned, "If this doesn't work, you'll have to have a cesarean!"

The mother didn't respond. She was so haggard, I don't think she cared at that point. In fact, she probably would have welcomed it as a relief from her nightmare.

2:35 A.M.—The rim of the cervix was still present and had thickened from the woman's efforts to push against it. Dr. Cox cut an episiotomy and started the vacuum extraction in spite of the cervical rim. I had to pump up the vacuum while he applied the suction cup to the baby's scalp (much like a bicycle pump).

"Pump it up harder!" he screamed at me.

2:45 A.M.—I sweated and struggled with the pump. Finally he took off the suction cup without even telling me. I suddenly noticed that there was no more resistance. I looked over to see that he had thrown it aside. The vacuum extraction was unsuccessful and he was preparing to repair the episiotomy.

As he sewed the episiotomy, he spotted a mole on the woman's labia. He finished the episiotomy and decided, since he was already there, to remove the labial mole. I thought he was joking. By then the baby's heart rate had already shown some signs of distress, and in the midst of all this, Dr. Cox decided to remove a labial mole! He cut it off and dropped it onto the sterile table with orders to send it to the lab in formaldehyde for analysis.

2:55 A.M.—While Dr. Cox called the operating room team to come up for a cesarean, we moved the mother from the birthing chair to the operating table. There was one small hitch to this. There was no electrical outlet near the operating table and the only way to adjust the birthing chair was electronically. We had to move a laboring mother, who was numb from the waist down, from a lower position in a birthing chair to a higher position on the operating table.

We finally pushed her onto the table and left her to labor there (on her back) while we set up for the cesarean. By now the epidural had worn off again, so she was screaming with every contraction. Dr. Cox was in the doctor's lounge now, ignoring her.

Meanwhile, back to the mole. As I wheeled the table out to the utility room, my aide had the formaldehyde prepared so I could just drop the mole in the jar. I picked up the mole with some tweezers and walked over to the jar. When I arrived at the jar, however, the mole wasn't in my tweezers—I had dropped it. It was precisely at that moment that we realized that the pattern on the floor was tiny flesh-colored spots on a black background. We immediately dropped to our knees to search for our lost mole.

What a sight we must have been, crawling all over the floor of the delivery room looking for our mole with a mother screaming on the operating table. The operating room team came crashing through the doors and screeched to a halt when they saw us on the floor. Luckily, we found the mole and saved ourselves injury from the stampede.

The operating room team had to replace the epidural because they said it was not put in appropriately. (Incidentally, no one was monitoring the baby this whole time, so if it had been in serious distress, no one would have known it.) While we were waiting for the epidural to be reinserted, Dr. Cox came to the nurses's station and asked me if I had ever "elevated" a baby's head during surgery. I looked confused as he explained. The excitement on his young boyish face reminded me of the Hardy Boys when they've solved a mystery.

"When I'm ready to take the baby out, I want you to put your fingers in her vagina and push the baby's head up," he said.

I looked at him in amazement.

He assured me that this was normal procedure as the baby's head would be too low for him to grab from the abdominal incision so I would have to push it up. He told me I would have to get used to it because it happens all of the time.

"Don't worry," he added, "I'll tell you exactly what to do and when."

The operating room team came out and announced that the mother was ready for us. I put on my sterile gloves and gown and waited to get my orders from Dr. Cox.

Suddenly, without warning, he yelled, "Okay, now!"

I jumped over to the operating table and pulled the mother's drapes off so I could get to her vagina. The operating nurses protested vehemently that I was contaminating the sterile field. (Dr. Cox hadn't warned them that I was going to do this.)

As I pulled the mother's drapes off I discovered that her legs were strapped together on the table and I had to pry them apart to get my hands in her vagina. The atmosphere was chaotic, with Dr. Cox screaming to hurry up and the nurses clumsily helping me after they realized that there was a method behind this madness.

I worked my hands between her thighs and attempted to put my fingers in her vagina as far as I could. Eventually, I worked my fist in there. I knew I would never forget this moment under the deep blue hue of the drapes.

My fingers brushed the obstetrician's as our hands met inside of our patient's pelvis. A nauseous feeling rose in my throat.

Miraculously, the baby boy did quite well, but the mother had to remain hospitalized for seven more days because she developed paralytic ileus, a condition where the intestines are temporarily paralyzed because of trauma during a surgical procedure. This is very painful as the abdomen becomes distended with trapped gas.

It saddened me to see her. Her body, once so wonderfully fit and supple, was now painfully swollen as she shuffled down the hall. She had to deal with an episiotomy, a cesarean, paralytic ileus and a new baby. She probably never noticed the stitches on her labia from the mole removal. Her motherhood and womanhood had been crippled. Her power had been stripped from her. I knew her intestines would heal shortly, but I wondered how long it would take for her psyche to heal.

The most frequent obstetric intervention I encountered was the use of drugs. In fact, it was rare that a patient went through the entire experience without drugs. Drugs were used for pain relief, to start or stop labors, to speed up labors and to slow them down. They were used to prevent women from lactating and to encourage them to have bowel movements. The most serious and most damaging of the drug use was for pain relief in labor. These drugs are the most serious because they have the potential to cause the most damage to the baby.

I suspect that some doctors ordered these drugs to make delivery easier on themselves. If the woman felt no pain, she was less demanding and could be easily ignored.

Dr. Pima administered a lot of drugs. One mother received two injections of 75 milligrams of Demerol (a potent narcotic pain reliever) during her five-hour labor. The last dose was one hour before delivery. Because Demerol severely blocks the baby's respiratory drive, the baby had to be resuscitated and was given a shot of Narcan (the antidote to Demerol).

Dr. Janson had a reputation for using Valium on his patients. I was told early in my tenure at the hospital that Dr. Janson required that we nurses carry a vial of Valium into the delivery room with us so that we could put it in the intravenous tube immediately after the baby was born. He didn't like to have a mother alert while he sewed up the episiotomy. He said they complained too much.

I didn't do too many deliveries with him, but when I did my first one, I purposely didn't bring the Valium in with me. Right after the baby was born, Dr. Janson asked for it. I said I didn't have it and walked out of the room to get it from the narcotics cabinet. I looked for the narcotics book to register my withdrawal and slowly walked back to the delivery room. By the time I came back, he had almost finished his suturing and I didn't need to give it. He was pretty mad at me.

"What took you so long?" he boomed.

"One of the other nurses had the keys to the narcotics cabinet," I answered.

"Well, she doesn't need it any more, but don't let this happen again," he warned as he threw his gown on the floor and walked out of the room.

Later I was in the recovery room with the woman helping her nurse the baby. The baby latched on quickly and nursed well. Because Valium can stay in the baby for eleven days, I'm glad the mother didn't have it. Also, she was awake to bond with an alert baby.

Dr. Janson's drug use was predictable. If any of his patients came in between 11:00 P.M. and 3:00 A.M., he ordered Nembutal, a potent barbiturate, so they would go to sleep. This way they would wait until morning to deliver. But a barbiturate depresses the baby as well as the mother, so if it doesn't work as planned and the mother doesn't stop laboring, she delivers a depressed infant who may not breathe. This doctor's habit of using narcotics was so well known that once during a continuing education seminar for nurses on infant resuscitation, the lecturer started her lecture with, "Now, when you're resuscitating Dr. Janson's babies. . . ." The audience laughed. Later, when she said that you can predict at least 50 percent of the babies that need resuscitation before they're born, one nurse piped up, "Yeah, just look and see if the patient is Dr. Janson's!"

A baby who doesn't breathe at birth loses vital oxygen to his brain. During my days as a teacher I had seen the long-term damage this could cause for the baby. I couldn't understand the arrogance of a doctor who dared to submit a baby to this danger just so he could get some more sleep.

One of the main reasons that drug use is so rampant in labor and delivery is that the mothers are so vulnerable at this time. They quickly follow the doctor's orders and ask for pain relief because they are scared of what is to come. They think that if the doctor says they're going to need it, they must need it. They know labor is going to hurt and they know they're going to be alone. The doctors have pushed the drugs for so long that some mothers come in demanding them. They've heard of the nightmare of labor from their mothers, their friends and their neighbors. Yes, labor is a nightmare in this system where women are left alone. The drugs are support substitutes.

Pain medications aren't the only drugs being pushed in maternity wards. The "labor manipulative" drugs are just as rampant. These are the drugs that speed up labor or slow it down. In other words, they tailor the labor.

Pitocin is a synthetic form of oxytocin, a powerful hormone in our bodies. Pitocin is by far the most widely used labor manipulative drug. It causes the uterus to contract. If the woman doesn't receive it before the birth to start contractions, make them stronger or speed them up, she receives it after the birth to prevent her from bleeding too much. (Encouraging the baby to nurse immediately causes the mother to release her own oxytocin in safer amounts.)

Just a few milliunits per minute, given intravenously, can cause the uterus to contract so violently that it can rupture and kill the fetus. Of course, there are now specialized machines that regulate the flow of pitocin intravenously, but it's not an exact science and it requires intense monitoring. Often hospital units are so understaffed that these pitocin drips are left unattended longer than they should be. More often than we would like to admit, these pitocin drips go awry creating fetal distress.

Dr. Voight had a woman come in ready to deliver twins. The babies were five weeks early and the mother's bag of waters had broken but she wasn't in labor. He decided to start a pitocin drip. (Given the research available, he probably should have waited as long as possible to induce labor because the babies were premature. Prematurity can result in many problems, including disability, cerebral palsy, and even death. The longer the babies had inside the mother's womb, the better.)

I was on evening shift. Dr. Voight called me from his office and ordered a pitocin drip at ten drops per minute.

Because of the risk of uterine rupture, our protocol said that we could only start with three drops per minute and then increase three drops every fifteen minutes until we got three contractions in ten minutes. I informed him of this rule.

"Well, with twin pregnancies you can start a little higher," he said.

"I'm sorry, Dr. Voight," I answered. "We're not allowed to administer pitocin at any dose that is higher than our protocols. You'll have to come do it yourself."

He was irritated. "Oh, all right," he snapped into the phone. "But be sure you have everything ready for me when I get there." He slammed down the phone.

He came over and started the pitocin at his dosage. Of course the uterus responded quickly and violently. The mother had a three minute contraction. (The baby doesn't get oxygen very well during contractions, so a contraction should never last longer than sixty seconds during a pitocin induction.) Dr. Voight quickly turned down the drip. That contraction stopped, but her uterus continued having long contractions even though he kept turning down the drip. It wasn't until the pitocin drip was down to three drops per minute (as prescribed in our protocols) that the uterus started contracting at an acceptable level.

But Dr. Voight didn't want to wait. It was highly likely that he was going to do a cesarean section on this woman because it is rare to do a vaginal delivery of twins. But he had promised her that he would do everything he could to try a vaginal birth. Consequently, when he confronted his patient he was in a tough position caught between the reality of twin births and the unfair promise he had made to her prenatally. So he stretched the truth. (I know this because I had been involved in the administering of the pitocin and I was in the labor room with the mother when the doctor arrived to discuss the situation.)

He told her that she'd been on the pitocin for a couple of hours and had *made no progress.* That because her bag of waters had broken, the babies' risk of developing infection was getting higher and higher as time went on. Also, the pitocin stimulation could be dangerous and might cause her uterus to rupture and her babies to die. After all of this, he went through the motion of asking her to choose between vaginal birth and cesarean section.

Of course, she was vulnerable. Quickly her mind made reason out of his words. Why go through all of this pain and risk her babies' deaths at the same time?

She delivered two very tiny, premature twins by cesarean section. They were transferred to the neonatal intensive care unit at the university hospital.

Are normal healthy infants safer born in the hospital than at home? That was becoming a serious question for me. Hospitals' obsession with paperwork and routine have made all of us less sensitive to each patient's needs, which seems particularly abhorrent when the issues of birth and death are concerned. In most cases, the patient does fine being ignored in such a system, but in unique cases, such as when someone's baby dies, our lack of sensitivity can be a tremendous problem.

The following story is a perfect example of that insensitivity. A fetus had died before labor began, so Dr. Cox put the mother on a pitocin drip to get her labor started. She labored for a long time and the active phase of labor was torturous. Imagine her desperation, going through all of this to deliver a dead baby. The nurses tried to stay with her as much as possible but other women were being admitted throughout the night, and we were trying to maintain order in this chaos. In fact the janitor was sick, so I had to mop the floors of the delivery room after each delivery.

The mother was screaming for pain relief, so Dr. Cox ordered Stadol (an analgesic) for her and he went to sleep in the doctors' lounge. When she began pleading for an epidural, I called the lounge and woke him up.

"It's too early to put in an epidural!" he snapped at me. "The baby's head's not deep enough into the pelvis."

However, just a few nights before, he sat with a patient and pushed the epidural on her early in her labor when she originally didn't want one. Now, a patient is screaming for one and he thought it was too early. I lost my professional cool.

I said, "In light of the torture that this woman is experiencing giving birth to a dead baby, I think that can be overlooked."

There was silence on the other line.

"All right," he sighed, "I'll be right there."

When he came back, I had everything ready for him. He started his procedure but the mother was struggling through the contractions and was quite hysterical. I tried to soothe her as best I could, but another doctor was calling me to assist with a delivery.

I heard Dr. Cox say, "Do you want this thing or not because if you do, you're going to have to cooperate with me!"

The sentence gave me a chill.

The baby was born soon afterward. I wasn't present for the delivery but I walked in soon after. The mother had given birth on the bed in the labor room. The dead baby was wrapped in a blanket at the end of the bed. The mother was crying as Dr. Cox sewed up her perineum.

Later in the morning, on my way out of the delivery room, I froze when I saw that someone had thoughtlessly placed the dead baby on the extra bed in the hallway. The blanket had fallen away from her. I was taken aback at the sight of her even though she looked peaceful. In the midst of such a busy and chaotic place, there was an aura of stillness around her. She was so beautiful and so lifeless at the same time. She was pale, and her abdomen had started to turn blue, like a large bruise.

As I was standing there, the nurses' aide came to help me "dispose of the body." We were both numb and exhausted from an unusually busy night. We put tags on her and measured her. Her body felt smooth and cold. The supervisor, Mrs. Harper, came back to instruct us.

"Now," she said authoritatively, "we have to wrap it up in linen and take it to the morgue."

I got a sheet out of the linen rack.

"Oh no!" Mrs. Harper exclaimed. "You shouldn't use a new clean sheet! You see, these just get thrown away. It's not worth it to put a new clean sheet on it!"

I was stunned at her insinuation. This baby, who had tried so hard to be perfect and fought for so long to hold on to life in the womb, wasn't even worth a clean new sheet?

But occasionally in our labor system, a unique person such as the nurse Lynn retains her sensitivity amidst the chaos of an overwhelmed health care system. Lynn was fed up with the callous practices displayed at this hospital. She didn't make a secret of her feelings so she was often at odds with Mrs. Harper, who was a bossy brittle woman. I admired Lynn for standing up for what she thought was right.

One night an anencephalic baby was born on Lynn's shift. Anencephalic babies have no skull and are severely deformed. This is one of the most difficult deformities to deal with because of the grotesque appearance of the baby. Their appearance has earned them the unfortunate name of "anencephalic monster." Their deformities are incompatible with life, and most anencephalic babies live only a few hours.

When Lynn came on shift, the baby had just been born so she went in to relieve the nurse who was in labor and delivery. The baby had been removed from the room before she arrived. The mother had hemorrhaged, so they were in labor and delivery longer than usual.

When they were finished, Lynn busied herself cleaning the delivery room and taking care of the mother in the recovery room. Later, while she was in the utility room washing some instruments, she spotted a pile of sheets on the counter and decided to clean them up as well. She filled the pail and grabbed the sheets to put them in the hamper. They felt heavier than usual. She juggled them in one arm and reached for some blankets with the other. Suddenly she heard a whimper coming from the sheets. When she opened them up, she found the anencephalic baby—still alive. Someone had thrown him in the utility room to die.

Lynn was in tears when she told me this. She was overwhelmed at the sight of this baby, who was so ugly yet so valiantly trying to survive against all odds. His body was cold from lying in the sheets on the stainless steel counter.

Lynn said she couldn't leave him. All she could see was his little soul struggling so hard to make it. She called Chris, the other nurse on duty. They were close friends. Lynn told Chris that she was taking off for the rest of the shift. The two nurses decided that if anyone asked, Chris would say Lynn went home sick. Chris assured her that she could handle the patients.

Lynn took a rocking chair to the utility room and held the little anencephalic baby until he died. She rocked him and sang him lullabies. She warmed the baby with her body.

After he died, Lynn went home. She told me later she spent the rest of the evening staring out of her window.

I admire health care professionals like Lynn who uphold the value and integrity of life in whatever form it decides to present itself. That is the true function of a nurse.

5

ANOTHER ASPECT of hospital delivery that really began to irk me was the callous and unnecessary forced separation between mother and baby. Frequently as I left my shift in the mornings and passed the nursery, the newborn boys would be getting circumcised, strapped to a table, their arms and legs held straight by velcro straps. They screamed throughout the operation. Afterward, the nurses would wrap them up and put them in the incubators where they cried themselves to exhaustion. I couldn't understand why they didn't bring the baby to the mother for comfort.

As health care professionals, we are obligated to value all human life and see it as worthy of care and protection, but in this hospital nursery that meant only monitoring the baby's vital signs and thermal environment. It meant taking him to the nursery immediately after birth to weigh and measure him, put in his eye drops and administer his Vitamin K shot, then leaving him in the warmer until the pediatrician could examine him (sometimes it would take hours before the pediatrician came). But when it came to soothing him, or giving him the human contact he so desperately needed, there wasn't time. The nurses just don't have the time. But the mother does.

A baby who stays with his mother has more opportunity to breast-feed. The more he breast-feeds, the more he encourages her milk to be produced so he gets enough fluids. It's nature's supply and demand system. The more he demands, the more milk is provided. And, breast milk is the mainstay of an infant's health. It provides all of the nutrients the baby needs for the first year of life. It has antibodies to protect him against chronic disease and respiratory illnesses. It protects against diarrhea, constipation and food allergies. And it enhances good tooth and mouth development.

The mother benefits too. When the baby nurses right after delivery, the nipple stimulation causes her body to release oxytocin, the natural form of pitocin, creating uterine contractions so she won't hemorrhage. There's no doubt about it, the mother and baby set-up is a perfect one. It's even life-saving. But in America, it's often considered secondary to the nursery routine.

The pediatricians would also do well to remember that they are there for the mothers and babies. There's no reason why a pediatrician can't examine a baby in front of the mother. It would be a wonderful opportunity to teach her how remarkable her new baby really is; how he can see her face, how he turns to suck in response to stroking his cheek and how he can grab with his feet. But it takes time to go from room to room and examine the babies under the mothers' watchful eyes. And, it might be awkward to have to answer the mother's questions.

These separationist routines can be dangerous especially if the hospital staff is insensitive to or has negative attitudes about breast-feeding.

One night when I worked in the nursery I learned that the combination of exhaustion and insensitivity can be a dangerous one. One baby was labeled a "crier" by the night head nurse. She told me that his mother wouldn't listen to a word they said. She was a problem patient and her baby suffered the brunt of it.

I took the baby to his mother to nurse at 1:00 A.M. The mother was in pain from the episiotomy and she had sore nipples. She was the type of person who dramatized her pain somewhat, but she wasn't unapproachable. I talked with her as she nursed, and she and her baby did well. When I took him back to the nursery, he started crying so I soothed him with the pacifier until I got called to labor and delivery. When I left at 2:00 A.M., the nursery nurses had their hands full with many crying babies.

When I came back at 4:30 A.M. this baby was crying ferociously and the nurse told me that he just wouldn't stop. I went over to his bassinet and picked him up. He had linen burns on his knees. Sometimes when babies cry really hard they actually get up on their knees and creep up the bassinet until their head hits the top rim. Unable to go any further, they continue to rub their knees in a creeping motion so that the friction of the sheets irritates the skin on their knees. I put him over my shoulder, and as I patted him on the back I realized he was running a temperature.

As I checked him with the thermometer, I started shaking inside. Up and up it went. I felt my heart pounding. My knees were giving out from under me. Finally his fever registered 103.4°F under his arm. I called the head nurse over. My voice felt like it was squeaking.

"Oh," the nurse said nonchalantly (as if it happens every day). "He's dehydrated."

She checked his blood sugar. It was twenty (normal is ninety).

"He's hypoglycemic. He needs sugar water. These breastfed babies just don't get enough!"

She fed him a few ounces of sugar water. I wrapped him and took him out to his mother. He didn't nurse very well, but his temperature was down to 100°F by the time he got back to the nursery. The nurses fed him more sugar water and got the temperature down to 99°F by the time I left.

The nursery staff wasn't alone in their negative attitude about breast-feeding. The postpartum nurses complained about babies nursing "on demand," and mothers in labor and delivery weren't encouraged to breast-feed immediately after birth even though we all knew it was better for mother and baby.

One woman arrived in labor at the beginning of the night shift. When I came in at 11:30 P.M. she was about three to four centimeters dilated. She was shaking all over and having a rough time. I could tell she was scared. Her husband watched helplessly. Dr. Horton checked her vaginally and told her she needed some medication to relax. Dr. Horton left to sleep in the doctors' lounge. The patient told me that she was scared of taking the medication but she didn't know what to do because the contractions were hurting so bad. I told her to wait out the next few contractions and I would stay with her. We breathed through them together. Her husband got involved and kept encouraging her, and I helped her change positions often. Luckily, I had no one else in labor so I could give her my full attention.

As the night wore on she was getting more and more confident. I got her up to the bathroom, and she leaned on her husband to walk around the room for a while before getting back into bed. I raised the head of the bed and lowered the foot so that it was almost as if she were sitting in a chair. She progressed nicely. At 6:13 A.M. she delivered a healthy baby girl in the birthing chair. Dr. Horton came in just to deliver the baby.

The mother was so proud of herself. She labored and delivered the baby without any drugs at all. What a boost of confidence it must have given her. I truly felt I had helped this family get started safely and happily just by being there and supporting the mother through contractions.

But there was a tough learning experience waiting for me. The mother was planning to bottle-feed her baby. I was so elated by her delivery that when I was unsuccessful in encouraging her to breast-feed, I was crushed. But then I realized that I can't get everyone to do things the way I think is best. Each mother has needs and feelings that I know nothing about. My job is to provide all of the information I can, but then I must let each woman make her own decisions and respect her for it.

I came to grips with my patient's decision to bottle-feed, but what really frustrated me were the events that followed her delivery. I believe that, had the environment been different, she would have chosen to breast-feed.

We routinely gave Deladumone (a powerful synthetic estrogen) to bottle-feeding mothers to dry up their milk. Because Deladumone is such a potent estrogen, and because it must be given within two hours after delivery, we had to give mothers the literature to read about its side effects before we administered it. The literature is pretty difficult to read and the side effects sound pretty scary. After they read the literature (while they were having contractions), we made them sign a consent form. They got the shot on the delivery table, right after their babies were born. (Now, these drugs are not given because they were found to be ineffective and linked to dangerous side effects.)

At 1:00 A.M. I gave the Deladumone literature to this mother and she expressed concern about the carcinogenic effects of the drug. I asked her if she would consider breast-feeding and she said she would. Her husband was mildly supportive. Because her labor progressed so quickly, I felt it was inappropriate to discuss breast-feeding. She was working so hard with her contractions that it seemed important to do only one thing at a time.

Because she never gave her consent to use Deladumone, it wasn't administered in the delivery room. When she went to the recovery room I struggled to get her baby back to her as soon as possible, but the nursery routine was so cumbersome that it was impossible to get the mother and baby reunited and it took longer than usual because it was change of shift. (It is unacceptable that important events such as mother-infant bonding are interfered with by such mundane events as shift change.) Eventually she opted to take the Deladumone.

The personnel in the hospital I worked in not only discouraged breast-feeding among their patients, but also among their employees who were breast-feeding. I was one such employee. I will never forget how I was treated on the maternity ward.

Dr. Voight had a patient who had developed eclampsia (a very serious disorder resulting from high blood pressure in the mother. In most cases, it is preventable through proper nutrition guidance). This case was so severe that the baby was delivered prematurely and the mother suffered temporary blindness from retinal detachment. She had to remain on medication after the delivery, which meant she could not breast-feed.

At the insistence of the mother, the hospital looked for a donor for breast milk for her baby. Because I was still breast-feeding Ahren, I agreed to be the donor. I willingly built up my milk supply by avid pumping and drinking high volumes of fluid. For two weeks I used the hospital's electric breast pump and pumped my breasts during all of my breaks and lunches. At the end of each day, I was able to leave eight ounces for the baby as well as have enough to feed Ahren. (By that time Ahren was a twenty-pound baby who was solely breast-fed with no supplements.)

Finally, the little baby went home with his mother and there was no more need for my milk. However, the problem with that was that my breasts had grown used to supplying far more milk than I needed and I couldn't go for very long before they would be painfully full. The day after the baby went home, I went to use the hospital's breast pump to relieve my aching breasts, but there was a sign on the pump that read, "Not for Employee Use." The head nurse of the nursery had put the sign there.

I was stunned. At that moment my milk let down and within seconds the front of my scrub suit was soaking wet. Milk was dripping out of my breasts and my stomach felt as if someone had slugged it. I broke down and cried from frustration.

I went to the head nurse and asked her for an explanation. She avoided my eyes and murmured something to the effect that if I used the pump, everyone else would want to use it. (At the time I was the only breast-feeding employee in the hospital.) I told her that because I was donating milk at her request, I felt it was reasonable for me to use the pump until my milk supply went back down.

But she was steadfast in her refusal. It took all I had to walk away with dignity. She had used me and gotten what she wanted. She literally milked me for all that she could get. She seemed a poor choice to work in the newborn nursery, setting policies for mothers and their babies.

I went in the lunch room and cried. Another nurse walked in and consoled me.

"Hey, I've got a great idea!" she said. "Wait a minute and I'll be right back!"

She ran out of the room and I composed myself as I waited for her return.

She came back with all sorts of tubing and other paraphernalia. We went to an empty patient room, put our heads together and devised a breast pump with tubing and a Y connector attached to my collection cup. I attached one end of the tube to the wall suction unit and regulated the amount of suction with my thumb on the Y connector. It was great. In fact, it was almost better than the electric breast pump.

I found a storage room near the newborn nursery that was filled with boxes and occasionally was used for an isolation room. It had a wall suction unit and it was very private. I happily settled myself among the boxes to pump. I gulped down my sandwich while I pumped.

The next day I returned to find a sign on the door of my new little pumping station that read, "This room is to be used for ISOLATION PUR-POSES ONLY. No pumping." I went out to the nursery to confront the head nurse again, only to learn she had left for vacation immediately after putting the sign up.

Luckily I went on night shift that week and found another wall suction in the birthing room which I used. The birthing room was a new concept at the time, so it was rarely used by physicians. Also, on the night shift there were fewer staff; therefore there was less chance that I would be discovered.

I wasn't daunted, but too many other mothers give up breast-feeding in hospitals and the workplace where there is no support for them to continue. Wherever childbearing women live and work there should be provisions made to encourage them to breast-feed their babies.

6

AMIDST ALL of the near catastrophes, blunders in care and disrespectful attitudes that I had to live with during my year at this hospital, there were a few bright spots. One of these was the childbirth education classes I taught. These classes were for couples who were planning to have their babies at home. I trained through an organization in California that was dedicated to informing couples about the birth process.

One of the couples in my class planned to have a home birth but ended up in the hospital where I worked because of a complication in her pregnancy. Sharon and Greg, who had a six-year-old daughter, were due to have their second baby on February 29.

When Sharon called me about my class, she said that she had some vaginal bleeding in her fourth month and an ultrasound showed placenta previa. (Placenta previa is a condition where the placenta is implanted very low in the uterus, below the baby's head, making vaginal delivery impossible.) She had accepted the idea of having a hospital birth, maybe even a cesarean, but she was excited when she called me because there was a possibility that the previa had resolved and she could have a home birth. (Often during pregnancy, placentas will migrate up to the top of the uterus making vaginal delivery possible.) She would have another ultrasound and if the previa had resolved, Laurie the CNM had agreed to attend the delivery at home. Dr. Voight was the backup doctor.

Sharon's ultrasound showed that the previa had resolved and she began taking my class and planning for a home birth, but two days before her due date, the baby turned breech. Laurie worried. There seemed to be too many things going against a home birth. The baby kept turning from breech to the head down presentation. Sharon started spilling a lot of sugar in her urine. She might have been developing gestational diabetes and her history of having large babies (her daughter was ten pounds eleven ounces) worried Laurie even more. She finally decided against attending the birth at home so I promised to go to the hospital with Sharon and Greg to be their support person.

Finally the day came for Sharon's baby to be born. She called me at 7:00

A.M. after she had been having contractions throughout the night. I waited. By 11:30 A.M., she was confused about her labor and didn't know whether to go to the hospital. I went out to her home to check her.

When I arrived, she had been out walking with Greg and she looked radiant. I could tell she was in early labor. I examined her and found she was four centimeters dilated. I told her to go to the hospital in at least two hours.

When I arrived for my shift, Sharon and Greg were already in the birthing room, and things were going smoothly. The two most supportive nurses were on shift. We couldn't have asked for things to go better.

As Sharon labored, I wiped her forehead and helped her breathe through her contractions. We also used such midwifery practices as hot compresses, perineal massage and gentle pushing. Greg rubbed her neck and encouraged her. I could see their bond as a couple strengthening. They were wonderful to watch.

Sharon progressed nicely. Their son was born amidst their hard work and wonderment. He was a beautiful testament to their love. He was nine pounds nine ounces. Because of the midwifery practices we had used, Sharon had no perineal tear.

I got to catch the baby because the doctor didn't make it in on time. Sharon's delivery made me realize that, with support and guidance, a woman can have a beautiful delivery no matter where she was.

Right after Sharon's birth I attended another beautiful birth in the birthing room. A couple came in with their first pregnancy. They were frightened but open to my suggestions. The mother came in asking for pain medication but she wasn't sure she was in labor. While we waited to make sure she was in labor I taught her how to breathe through her contractions. Her husband was very supportive and kind. Their relationship seemed mature and loving.

They labored well together. He was able to encourage her while he, too, was going through an amazing life transformation. When he seemed to be unsure of himself, I stepped in to encourage him. The mother labored as a woman who loved her body. Once her initial fear was gone, her inner strength glowed. She had faith that her body would bring forth a miracle.

I kept using encouraging words. "You are strong. You are one contraction closer. You can do it," I kept repeating.

I got her up and walked her. I put her on the toilet reasoning that the position one takes on the toilet, upright and slightly squatting, would encourage her baby to descend and her cervix to dilate. I was correct, and she became completely dilated in one hour. I put her back on the bed and cranked the head up so she could be in a sitting/squatting position. (Gravity is a laboring woman's best friend.)

When their baby was born, the father was euphoric and swore he saw a glow around the baby. It was love at first sight, which is the way it should be.

On night shift I was pretty much alone on labor and delivery. I had either a licensed practical nurse or an aide who worked with me, but if we had a woman in labor, I usually was in the room with them so my aide wandered to another section of the floor to chat with the nurses.

It was nice being on night shift because the doctors would rather sleep than hassle me. Being left to my own devices, I developed a few techniques to help women through labor. My most infamous one was the toilet. I put every woman I could on the toilet with a pillow behind her back. Their husbands would sit in front of them on the floor. I put a cup of ice next to them on the sink so husbands could wet their wives' lips to quench the thirst of labor. When I had two or more women in labor, I got as many as I could up on the toilets and I scurried back and forth to support and monitor them.

I developed a reputation for getting the babies delivered faster than others. Once Dr. Horton was walking down the hall telling the nurses that he would be at home if they needed him. One of his patients was in labor. As I passed him in the hall to report for shift, he changed his mind and said that I could call him in the doctors' lounge. He was tired of missing the births on my shift.

One night when one of Dr. Voight's patients was in labor I had her on the toilet almost my entire shift. She had arrived in labor two shifts before and Dr. Voight was considering a cesarean because of her lack of progress. When I came in she was at her wit's end. I got her onto the toilet and tactfully suggested that she stay there for a few contractions. She agreed. In fact, she liked it so much that she decided to stay there.

Much to my dismay, Dr. Voight came in to check her at 4:00 A.M., and he caught us in the bathroom. I couldn't say that she was urinating because her husband was sitting on the floor in front of her and I was perched on the sink. She had a pillow behind her back and was breathing beautifully through her contractions.

He insisted that she get in the bed so he could do a vaginal exam to decide whether to do a cesarean. To his surprise, he discovered that her cervix was completely dilated and she was ready to push her baby out. He instructed her to push. She made no progress after one hour of pushing while she was lying on her back, so he decided that we should take her to the delivery room to see if she would push better on the delivery table. Still no progress.

Finally, he looked at me in exasperation and said, "Why don't you find the bedside commode and bring it in here. We could have her push on that and maybe the baby's head will come down."

I happily brought it into the delivery room. His patient sat on the commode to push and her baby was born fifteen minutes later.

I felt wonderful after these births. My need to become a midwife became more prevalent. I loved this work and felt I was helping women become mothers in a peaceful, healthy and dignified way. I was convinced these babies were being born with gentleness, love and comfort, which made them happy and strong so that they could put all of their energy into bonding instead of trying to keep warm and safe.

In early May I found out that I was on the waiting list at the School of Midwifery of Georgetown University. If no positions opened I wouldn't make it in. Eric eased my depression with a midnight plan in early June. "Juliana," he said quietly as he shook me awake. "We need to move."

I turned to him, my eyes groggy with sleep. "Where?" I asked wearily. We had just moved to this duplex less than a year ago and I had grown tired of being so unsettled.

"Somewhere closer to Georgetown," he answered.

I was wide awake now.

"Look," he reasoned. "You're first on the waiting list. What if they call you right before school starts? If we live way down here, we won't be ready to go at a moment's notice."

This would mean I would have to quit my job at the hospital. "What will we live on?" I asked.

"It's simple," he assured me. "I'll get a job as a speech pathologist in the public schools in a neighboring county and if they call you, we'll already be there and settled."

His plan was so reasonable. I knew it was what we had to do. He gave me hope. The move would symbolize a commitment to move forward.

Within a week he got a job. I gave a month's notice at work.

My last day at work was drab and boring. Eric called me to say that Ahren had diarrhea. No one was in labor so I went home early. I cleaned out my locker and gave my jacket to one of the other nurses. I walked out, accidentally leaving behind my nursing shoes. I guess I was subconsciously planning never to be a nurse in a hospital again.

7

FINALLY August 30 rolled around. It was the day of registration for midwifery school. Even Eric lost hope that I would be accepted. Somehow, I had a final surge of optimism . . . maybe someone wouldn't show up.

I reconciled myself to my schedule. I was a part-time student registered for two courses, statistics and nursing concepts. At least I'd have time for Ahren and could accept a part-time job.

Registration was depressing. I looked around at the six women who had gotten accepted to the midwifery program. What did they have that I didn't?

The next day started out peacefully. In fact I was pretty content. I accepted the change in my master plan. I decided to be productive. I sent my children's story to a magazine to see if they would publish it. I even did the finances for September.

In the evening I got the kids to bed and by 9:00 P.M. was satisfied I would live until next year when I was assured a place in the program.

At 9:15 P.M. the phone rang. It was the chairman of the midwifery department at school.

"Hi, Juliana? How are you?" she started.

"Fine, how are you?" I answered. I was curious. Why was she calling me so late? I started to worry. Maybe they decided that they didn't want any part-time students after all. Maybe she was going to tell me to forget about coming. I sat down.

"What are you doing tomorrow?" she asked.

"Nothing much," I answered, my voice shaking. "Why do you ask?"

"Well," she started out haltingly. "Our grant came through tonight at 6:00 P.M. We've been meeting ever since and we decided that we want you and the next student in line to start school full-time tomorrow. I'm not positively sure that things are going to work out, but I'm 95 percent sure. I will be sure at about 11:00 tomorrow, but I want you to start orientation tomorrow with the rest of the full-time students."

By the time she finished her sentence, I had slid off my chair and laid down on the cold kitchen floor. I could hardly breathe. Now I knew what it meant to be "floored." This was the call for which I had been waiting for two years. This was it! This was it! But, was I really in? I couldn't believe I was in!

"Juliana? Are you there?" the chairman called into the phone.

I couldn't speak. Eric almost grabbed the phone from me.

"Yes, I'm here," I gasped into the phone.

The chairman giggled. She realized what was going on. She had patiently put up with my badgering for two years and she knew how much this meant to me.

"Can you be there tomorrow at nine?" she asked.

"Definitely," I answered.

I don't remember what I did when I hung up. Everything from that point on is a blur. I had diarrhea all night. I borrowed two cigarettes from a neighbor and smoked them on the front steps in the middle of the night.

The next morning I dropped the children off at a friend's house. She could keep them for the day. Somehow I made it to the school and walked into the room where orientation was held. I spent the first two hours wondering whether I would be in or out. I found the woman who was on the waiting list after me. We stuck together like peas in a pod.

At 11:00 A.M. we stopped for a break. The other student and I were standing in the hall when the department chairman walked up with tears in her eyes.

"You're in!" she said as she gave me a hug.

At that moment I left one ordeal and entered another. I was officially a student nurse-midwife!

I had entered school thinking that all the midwifery students would be like me and that we would unite and conquer. But I was wrong. We were a divergent group with very different reasons for choosing this path. Later, I would learn that we would not automatically support each other. Rather, our struggle to form a cohesive group would be long, difficult and an ongoing process. Many pitfalls would stand in our way; particularly burnout and the persuasiveness and power of technological obstetrics.

Looking around the group that first day, I could not have determined what each individual's motives were for being there, though in my usual way, I made snap judgements that proved to be wrong. I would learn that Lisa, who seemed so flaky, was in fact really quite serious, and she and I shared similar philosophies about home birth, nonintervention and no medication during labor. And there was Abbey, who I immediately decided was insolent. But I would later discover that it was she who brought our diverse group together. I would discover that Cathy wanted a very conservative practice with a physician. Hospital birth was definitely the only thing for her. And there was Patty, who annoyed me the first day because she seemed concerned that registration was going to get in the way of her hair appointment. Patty would become my very favorite person in the program. Her demeanor seemed to emanate from her appearance and she would change hair color throughout the year. No wonder her clothing, hair and make-up seemed important; they added to her vibrancy, positive attitude and fresh approach to the world, which would ultimately make her the special midwife she would become.

I would learn the most valuable lesson in school from these classmates: Midwifery is an art. We are professionals, but just as you can't have two professional painters paint on the same canvas, you can't expect two midwives to manage a labor the same way. What we learned in school were skills. How we used those skills was the art.

There were eight students and six faculty members, two of whom were just about the same age as myself. After the faculty introduced themselves, our program director spoke, saying even the students should consider ourselves midwives already, that we were all equal in the program, student and faculty. She emphasized that we had all chosen to walk the same path together, and that we must support each other so that by the end of the program, we would all be richer. Her words brought tears to my eyes. Ever since that sunny afternoon six years before when I had known I was a midwife, I had been trying to prove to everyone that it was so. Finally, I was being recognized as one. I glowed inside.

There was much work ahead. The curriculum was divided into modules: health assessment, antepartum (prenatal), intrapartum (labor and delivery), postpartum (after delivery), gynecological (women's health care), neonatal (newborn), professional issues, and patient education. We could go through the modules at our own pace, but we had to be finished by a certain deadline. At the end of the deadline we had to take an all-day essay exam in which we had to make a 95 or we would flunk. We had the chance to take the test once more. The re-test would be oral and it could be on anything in the module, not necessarily the things we got wrong.

Each module consisted of questions that we had to answer through research in the library from the most current information available worldwide. When completed, each module could be expected to be over one hundred and fifty pages long. All of that information had to be memorized.

The modules were the core of our curriculum. Our courses and clinicals were complementary to them. In addition to the modules, there were courses in business management, research, and business administration.

As we sat huddled around that table on orientation day in a large auditorium listening to our instructors, I looked around at my classmates' faces and saw that they were expressionless. I was terrified. Could it be that they had a handle on things so quickly? They didn't look as overwhelmed as I felt. Suddenly I realized that I had spent so much of my energy trying to get into school that I had not even thought about getting through school. I felt like a bride who put so much of her time into her wedding that she didn't take the time to consider how she was going to make it through the marriage. I was frightened. I felt as if I were suffocating. I did everything to keep my panic at bay. It was the first of many times in the following years that I would feel this way. I learned quickly to do what I told my laboring women: breathe deeply and evenly, and above all, relax.

In the fall semester, we started antepartum care. A precedent to this module was the health assessment module where we learned to do physical exams. Through this training I developed a sense of what the rest of the year was going to be like. My fascination with the human body was renewed. I came home with a sore pelvis every day while we practiced on each other, learning to do pelvic exams. Needless to say, this module did nothing for my sex life.

The fall semester was crazy. We were doing prenatal clinics at H.P. General Hospital (HPGH) and City Wellness Association (CWA). I remember feeling confused most of the fall. I felt like I never put things together in an integrated way. I was too busy memorizing what blood tests patients needed and what the differences were between HPGH and CWA protocols for lab work.

I remember my first day at CWA. I arrived to meet Rhonda, the midwife I would observe that morning. She was a Yale graduate and about five months pregnant. I wasn't too thrilled with the environment. I don't know what exactly I thought midwifery practice would be—homey furnishings and long discussions with patients—but this wasn't it. All I saw were white lab coats, paper exam tables, bland metallic offices, and patients coming in and going out in fifteen-minute intervals. I was beginning to learn that there were many forms of midwifery.

The day proved to be long. By its end my breasts were aching and I was exhausted. I pumped out my milk in the bathroom, saved it and started the long commute home.

The next day we had our orientation at HPGH. Cheryl, a part-time faculty member, oriented us. She was nice but HPGH was a substandard facility in the inner city. The nurses at first seemed cooperative, but they were putting on a nice show. I had already heard that they didn't like having the midwives around. Our indoctrination was fast and hard. Behind the smiles were sneers and eyes filled with contempt. These nurses were hardened by seeing the most difficult kind of patient and the most inexperienced health care provider. There was nothing they hadn't experienced: heroin addiction in mothers and their babies, multiple drug abuse, murder victims, and psychiatric cases.

On top of that they had to put up with troops of medical residents and student nurse-midwives. New people constantly, coming into their environment, shouting out orders that they had to follow. Often the nurses knew more than we did. To stand by watching all of us make mistakes must have been frustrating for them. Sometimes they would tell us the orders we should be giving.

HPGH prenatal clinic was truly a cultural shock. It was like welfare row. Poor women, mostly black and Hispanic, were crowded into a small waiting room. To this day I still see their faces. Their expressions seemed a sad combination: scared, defiant, and indifferent.

One day a woman came into the clinic with a little girl who was about three years old. The little girl was playing and making the nice natural noises that children make, but the woman had a belt around her hand and was constantly threatening to use it on her. I was horrified. I went to the director of the HPGH midwifery service, and told her that I thought we should report her to child protective services. She said that it wouldn't help and to forget about it. I was to learn that often, when you work with this population, you become resigned to small abuses. Sometimes the art is to know where to draw the line between small abuses and large abuses.

A few days later during prenatal clinic, I had a patient who was twenty-one years old, having her first baby. I was getting a little better at asking medical histories. She told me that she was newly pregnant and hadn't felt the baby move yet. (Usually an expectant mother will feel her fetus move around the fourth to fifth month.) After I asked her all of the questions, I began to muddle my way through her physical exam. Basically, in a physical exam, you start at the head and work down. Cheryl, my instructor, was in the room observing me.

I made it through her exam without any problems until I got to her abdomen. When I uncovered her abdomen, I could see that she was quite pregnant. I could even see the baby kicking. I stopped in confusion. She told me that she was newly pregnant. How could this be? I looked at Cheryl, but she shrugged her shoulders as if to say, "You're in this alone." This was, after all, my clinical training.

The mother looked at me and said, "What's wrong?"

"Well," I stammered, "I think you're much more pregnant than you think you are."

"What do you mean?" she asked me in alarm.

"From your size and the fact that I can see your baby moving, I think you're going to have this baby sooner than you think," I answered.

I felt my body get clammy with perspiration. I was feeling unsure about what I was saying, but I measured her abdomen. "You're about seven months pregnant," I told her.

The mother broke down and cried. Apparently, she wanted this baby to be fathered by the boyfriend she had now rather than the boyfriend she had seven months before.

I comforted her. Now, I surely hoped that I was right. I would hate to get a thrashing and have caused this woman so much anguish on top of it.

Somehow I got through the rest of the exam. It wasn't easy with a tearful patient and a watchful instructor. I didn't know where I stood. I wrote up the report and left the room with Cheryl. The cool air of the hallway felt refreshing. We walked the mother over to the lab to get her blood drawn for tests. All the while I was worried that I had made a terrible mistake. Cheryl wasn't giving a sign at all.

Finally we were alone. I knew it would start.

"That was a great job you did in there, Juliana!" Cheryl exclaimed. "I'm really proud of you. It's really hard to be told one thing in the history and find something that totally contradicts that in the physical."

I felt all of my insecurity come bubbling to my lips as my tension struggled to be released. I stopped myself from letting her know what I was thinking. "No, Juliana," I cautioned myself. "Act confident."

I thanked her and, sighing with relief, I hurried on to my next patient.

My prenatal clinic at CWA was totally different from HPGH. CWA was the "doctor's office" routine. The patients were all middle class, employed people.

It was at CWA that I started to get the hang of things: my knowledge and skills started to come together and I learned to follow the format as I went along. Time constraints were strict: one hour for the first prenatal visit, one half hour for the first gynecological visit, and fifteen minutes for everything else except one half hour for an occasional teaching visit. I hoped I could give the women personalized care. I tried to fill out the forms and stay within the time limits, a feat that I could barely accomplish even by the end of the semester.

On the other end of the spectrum, my clinical at HPGH for labor and delivery consumed me physically, emotionally, and philosophically. I quickly learned to cope by shutting my eyes to the flagrant abuses of human dignity that happened daily in that hospital. I was too busy, too tired, and too involved with getting through school with a remnant of sanity. I couldn't take on any causes.

My self-centered feelings made me understand (but not condone) the apathy of the residents there. Their rotations are so demanding. Their hours are ungodly and often they go days with no rest. I felt sorry for them and worried about patients for whom they made decisions after being deprived of sleep for so long. These young doctors struggled to make it through the day while suffering from sleep and food deprivation.

When I had been finally accepted into the program, I called my parents, and my mother arranged to fly to America. She arrived the day after Labor Day and stayed throughout my program to be with Ahren while I was in school. I was thankful to have my mother who not only took care of Ahren but also of me.

I couldn't have done this program if it hadn't been for my mother. Although she was slightly incapacitated with Parkinson's disease, she restored order to my home and had dinner waiting for me in the evenings. She made sure that we all stayed healthy during the following year and a half. She was there to see Anneke off to school and waiting for her when she got home. She held Ahren as I waved good-bye to both of them in the morning. She faithfully fed him my breastmilk with a cup and made it possible for me to continue breastfeeding. My mother was my backbone. It is due to her that I can give other mothers and babies all the care that I do.

Because of my wonderful, supportive family, things at home were going as smoothly as possible. Eric loved his job. He never complained about work or about my hours, but I could tell that the stress of my school was taking its toll on him. His psoriasis was not doing very well. He went to a dermatologist who prescribed some cortisone-saturated tape to apply to his psoriasis patches every night. At first the condition improved, but as the fall semester wore on, I noticed it was getting worse again and he was putting the tape over more and more of his body.

My father came to visit in November and temporarily relieved my guilt about separating my mother from my father. However, it was obvious that my mother, in spite of her Parkinson's disease, was thriving at feeling functional again.

Christmas vacation was long awaited for. The antepartum module had been difficult. There was a wealth of information to learn and integrate. The final exam was an essay that took eight hours to complete. We all had to take the oral re-tests.

Somehow, the work didn't seem like the hard part. Sometimes it seemed like it took more effort to deal with the people than the school. My classmates were intense and competitive. Most were more group oriented than I.

My focus was highly individual. I had tunnel vision. I had a heavily regimented schedule to which I felt I needed to adhere to survive. Every morning I woke up, nursed Ahren and jumped out of bed. I immediately made the bed, made my mother's bed, and dressed the children. I brought Ahren down with his diapers for the day.

I didn't want my mother to go upstairs frequently throughout the day because of her Parkinson's disease. If she fell, there would be no one around to help her.

After breakfast I would leave for my one and a half hour commute to school. I made tapes of my notes so I could listen to them on the way.

On days when I had no classes or clinicals I studied at home. Because it was hard for me to study with Ahren climbing all over me, my mother and I developed a great system. After breakfast, I would drive away as if I were going to school. My mother would stand in the door holding Ahren and they would both wave good-bye to me. Then, she'd take him into the living room and I would drive around to the back of the house. While she kept him occupied, I would sneak back into the house and keep myself locked in the upstairs room for the day. Ahren never knew I was home. My mother quickly brought lunch up to me, and at 5:00 P.M. I would walk down the stairs. He never caught on to our trick. By the end of fall semester I had settled into my role as a student nurse-midwife.

It was shortly after the spring semester began that I delivered my first baby as a midwife. It was one of the first days of the semester and we weren't delivering babies yet, but the director of the midwifery department at the hospital poked her head into the room to say they were extremely busy in delivery and were we interested in helping out. At first the entire room was quiet. Then I jumped at the chance and Lisa followed suit and before we knew it, we were hustled up to the floor. Jamie, our chairperson, came with us.

There were women in labor everywhere. The rooms were filled and some patients were out in the hallways. No one was monitoring them. I was pushed into a room with a Hispanic woman who spoke no English.

Lisa and Beth took over because they were both fluent in Spanish. Just about then another woman in labor was admitted and there was havoc. Everyone was running around like chickens with their heads cut off. Sometimes hospitals are screwy to the point where they're unsafe.

"Where can we put her?" someone implored.

The delivery room and labor rooms were full. It was obvious that this woman was going to deliver her baby imminently.

"Over there!" someone cried pointing to the supply desk.

"No! Over there!" someone else cried.

They finally pushed her into a patient's room, which meant the original laboring occupant had to be sort of shoved over. Wonderful, assertive Jamie recognized a chaotic situation that she could use to our advantage. She grabbed me and pushed her way into the room with the new occupant. Before I knew it, I was delivering the baby. It came out with the bag of waters intact. I popped the bag of waters and out came the head. I was so proud of myself because amid all the chaos I remembered to check for a cord around the neck. Looking back, what I remembered is that instead of finding a cord, I grabbed hold of the baby's hand. It seemed as though he was trying to climb out. Soon there was a brand new seven pound, twelve ounce beautiful baby boy in the world. His mother experienced a very small perineal tear and I sewed it up myself. Jamie stood next to me and coached me through. It was hard to see through my tears. Birth is so beautiful. I was ecstatic. (A few days later I heard that Jamie was criticized by the HPGH staff because she didn't change out of her black boots for the delivery.)

I'll never forget my second delivery. The mother was a twenty-six-year-old Hispanic woman having her first baby. Her labor progressed beautifully and three and a half hours later she gave birth to a little girl. For the delivery, she was flat on her back with her legs in the stirrups. At HPGH, all women who delivered in the delivery room had to be in this position, called the lithotomy position, which has been documented to prolong pushing time and lead to more perineal lacerations. The lithotomy position is good for only one person, the birth attendant, because it makes the perineum accessible for episiotomies and forceps deliveries.

The position, however, puts mother and baby at a severe disadvantage. The woman does not have gravity to help her and she must push harder. When she pushes harder and uses brute force to deliver her baby, she loses touch with the messages in her body that tell her to slow down, stop pushing, and deliver her baby gently. A gentle delivery protects the mother's perineum from tearing. The lithotomy position also necessitates that the attendant take more control, commanding the mother to push hard to overcome the loss of gravity's help.

Midwives believe in the integrity of the bodies of both the mother and baby. If needed, a midwife will do an episiotomy, but it is our conviction that tissues that weren't torn or cut heal better and less painfully than tissues that must form scar tissue in an attempt to recapture their previously healthy state. Many M.D.'s, on the other hand, encourage the mother to push with all of her might and then they cut an episiotomy. The baby's head pops out quickly, often causing the episiotomy to tear further into the mother's anus and rectum.

As my patient pushed, I was involved in setting up my table, lining up my cord clamps, scissors, syringe with lidocaine (in case I had to make the cut). The baby was coming slowly so I thought I had plenty of time. My instructor was telling the mother to pant to ease the baby out slowly.

Suddenly my instructor cried out, "Watch out!"

Out popped the baby's head. I saw the mother's perineum burst right before my eyes. It was like a race car bursting through a paper billboard at the finish line. I still cringe at the thought.

We spent the next one and a half hours sewing up a huge tear. I put in a pudendal block to numb her perineum so she wasn't feeling any pain, but I felt sad that she had to spend the time flat on her back with us sewing her up rather than with her baby. I learned a valuable lesson: Don't ever stop watching the perineum when the baby's head is crowning.

My next birth was with the same instructor. We had taken to roaming the halls of HPGH after each birth. There was a lot going on in labor and delivery, but there were many medical students and residents so no one was willing to turn a patient over to us. Besides, if we just had a delivery, we were "third up," meaning, we would get the third low-risk patient admitted to the hospital. (Sort of like shoe salesmen in a department store rotating turns at customers.)

Often I had taken these roaming times as an opportunity to observe the management of complicated, high-risk deliveries. I figured the more I watched, the more I would learn. And, since I was "handy," it was often convenient for one of the residents to ask for my help. I got a lot of hands on experience that way.

On this particular day, there was a woman laboring in one of the rooms who was having her eighth baby. She was pretty low-risk so the residents were leaving her alone while they were handling other cases. They had put a medical student in the room with her to keep an eye on things. He was sitting in the farthest corner of the room looking pretty lost. In fact, he was looking petrified at the possibility that, since no one was around, he might be put in the position of delivering the baby alone. (Amazingly, medical students don't necessarily have to do any deliveries while they do their obstetric rotation.)

Cheryl said, "Go show that student that it doesn't take years of schooling to know that sometimes the best kind of health care you can give is a back rub and a few kind words of encouragement. And be ready to catch that baby. Those eighth babies come out quick. I'll be down in the nurse's lounge. Call me if you need me."

The mother was Hispanic, so I struggled with my few rudimentary Spanish words but I had learned quickly that the language of caring is universal. She smiled at me with appreciation as I started to rub her back. She rested her hand on my arm and squeezed it gently every time she felt a contraction starting. Within minutes we had quite a communication system going. I motioned for the medical student to move closer. He smiled at me and pulled his chair up to the bed. He watched intently as we continued with her labor.

Suddenly her eyes flew open with that look that could only mean one thing. The baby was coming. She was on her side so I lifted her leg to check. Sure enough, there was the baby's head sliding out. I called for help and implored her not to push. The baby virtually dropped into my hands.

Everyone came running. The first one in was the head nurse who looked at me accusingly. "I heard you tell her to push!" she said.

"That's not true," I returned, "I told her not to push!"

"I heard you say, 'Push! Push!' " she sneered.

Deciding to ignore her, I placed the baby on the mother's chest. Luckily the two got to be together longer as the nurses ran around looking for instruments to cut the cord. I even got the baby to breast-feed before they came back. I took as much time as I could to cut the cord so no one could take the baby away. The medical student remained beside the bed, standing as if he was protecting us from the onslaught of onlookers. After everything was over he went to the head nurse and told her that I was indeed telling the woman not to push.

I was bewildered by the head nurse's reaction. It was as if she was accusing me of stealing the patient from the residents.

I *do* understand some of the negative feelings nurses have toward midwives and residents. After all, new student midwives and residents are constantly coming through the hospital, and nurses have too many people giving them orders. I'm sure that I would eventually resent a sea of faces treading over my terrain, barking orders and leaving the area trampled. And a hospital truly can be a safety hazard with broken monitors, lost emergency carts and filthy admitting rooms. The students' stays there are temporary, so they don't have the motivation to clean it up. And the permanent staff is too tired.

Unfortunately, it's really the mothers and babies who suffer. Most often a woman is left alone to labor, lying flat on her back. No one rubs her back or helps her change positions. No one gets her up to urinate. And when she desperately calls for help, no one listens. Just as long as she has a fetal monitor around her, she's receiving the "best care."

Large modern teaching hospitals are there for the students. In the obstetrical area, the only way to handle the patient load and give all the students an opportunity to learn is to treat the labor area like an assembly line. Each laboring woman is a "case" and the student goes from case to case taking from it all that can be learned. As the woman moves down the assembly line from the admitting office to labor and delivery, her labor is subject to more and more obstetrical intervention. The students must learn how to master the technology.

As the woman's labor picks up in emotional intensity, she cries out in fear, pain, frustration and exhaustion. In an assembly line, because there is no time for emotional expression, there is no tolerance. Her cries are merely indicators that she needs pain medication. This is convenient because the residents must learn how to administer it.

If the mother's labor isn't knocked out by drugs, her "fight or flight" response is activated and reactivated and the effects of the continued release of adrenaline take hold: the blood vessels are constricted for hours and the blood flow to the uterus eventually is compromised. This, in combination with making her lie on her back (which cuts off circulation) and withholding nourishment for hours (even days), can make the uterus stop working effectively and her labor takes longer. And on and on it goes.

In this situation, the student leaves each case in the assembly line smarter; one step closer to getting the expertise needed to make it in the high-tech world of obstetrics. The mother, though, is not as fortunate. The failure cycle has begun. It will be perpetuated in a variety of ways and by the time she bundles the baby up to go home, it will have taken hold. And even though the student has succeeded, his success is fragile because as long as the mother feels a sense of failure, we all fail. Ultimately, it is the success of the mother that is most important because the mother is the cornerstone of any society.

In order to avoid falling into the assembly line mentality, my classmates and I knew we needed to take care of ourselves during spring semester, so we started weekly group counseling. We did this at the suggestion of a previous class who thought it helped them get through school. It was here that I learned some new things about myself and how I appeared to other people. I began to tackle my feelings of fear of losing, which come across as competitiveness. I had entered every difficult situation in my life assuming I would lose and fighting not to. Now, I began to learn how to tackle challenges with more confidence. As my midwifery education continued, this understanding of the need to partner with others rather than win or lose became extremely important.

As the weeks of school went on, we mastered our midwifery skills, taking care of mothers, delivering babies, and providing gynecological and contraceptive care to women of all ages. During that time I had clinicals at CWA, HPGH, and a family planning center in Baltimore.

Even though my days were grueling, I enjoyed these clinicals. I saw patients all day who came from a variety of settings.

One day while I was at CWA, a woman came in for her annual exam. She had a daughter who was six years old and she and her husband were trying to conceive a second child, but they weren't having any success. They were considering getting some help from fertility experts. I saw the opportunity to do a preliminary fertility workup.

I started asking her the regular questions about her menstrual cycle in the past and present, her past medical history, family history, and so on. Then, because fertility takes two, I asked her some of the same questions about her husband. After those questions, I had to get more personal: Are there any problems at home? How much alcohol/cigarettes/drugs do you or your husband consume? Then much deeper: Tell me about your sexual practices, especially frequency of intercourse.

I couldn't believe the answer I got. "Well, we have intercourse about once a month," she said. "Sometimes we miss a month."

"Once a month!" I said to her, "That's pretty infrequent if you want to conceive a child."

I went on to explain a little bit about the menstrual cycle and how it was important to have intercourse during the fertile times in the cycle. I quickly saw that I needed to start from the beginning. She had absolutely no idea what I was talking about. I made a mental note to have her come back for a teaching appointment so I could give her more information. Because I only had a half hour to spend with her (and I still had to do her physical exam), I left my advice simple: "Have intercourse more frequently and you will increase your chances of becoming pregnant."

When I did her physical exam, I saw that she had a lot of fertile mucus coming from her cervix and I quickly calculated that, with her menstrual cycle, this could definitely be a fertile time for her. I showed her the mucus and told her that this might be a good time to have intercourse. I think she took me literally because after her appointment was over she told me that she was going to call her husband and have him come home from work immediately. I gave her directions to the pay phone downstairs and never heard from her again. Maybe the family planning worked.

Anne, one of the residents I worked with at HPGH, was in her last tri-mester of pregnancy. She seemed to be a very kind woman but distant as she attempted to push her increasingly bulky body through her rotations. During one night shift she was particularly busy and toward the end of the shift, a woman arrived in labor with twins. The woman had had a previous cesarean, so the plan was to do a repeat cesarean. Because she was in labor, the oper-ation couldn't wait until the next shift.

Because Anne was the chief resident on duty and the other residents were busy with other cases, she had to do the cesarean herself. Anne had been up for thirty-six hours. Her feet, face and hands were puffy. I finished with two deliveries and I was on my way out of the hospital when I found her trying to call an escort who could go with her to bring the patient's lab work to the lab. The residents at HPGH are required to take the lab work down themselves. And because of recent crimes in the hallways, an escort was needed whenever you had to walk any distance in the hospital.

Anne looked beaten to the limits as she waited on the phone. The lab was far away from labor and delivery, so the walk was not only dangerous, but long. Meanwhile, her patient was starting to scream with her contractions. Time was becoming more of a factor. Anne couldn't wait for the escort. I offered to walk with her just to make sure that she would make it there and back.

She was quiet as she shuffled through the halls. I could tell her back was hurting and her feet were aching. I felt like putting my arm around her so she could lean on me. I tried talking to her, but she just smiled at me sadly and continued on her way. She was probably too tired to move her jaws. I felt so sorry for her: not only did she have to make this journey, but she had to do a cesarean to deliver twins when she got back. I also thought of the welfare of her patient. I'd never go under the knife of a person who hadn't slept for thirty-six hours. I stayed with her through the operation, after which she was relieved by another resident.

After watching doctors go through grueling residencies, I understood one reason why they charged a lot of money in their practices—they went through hell to get their degrees and they felt like they deserved to be rich.

Well into the spring semester, I was doing a newborn exam "on the sly" as I visited a mother and her infant on postpartum rounds. At HPGH, nurse-midwives had to do newborn exams clandestinely because we were forbidden by the head physician of the newborn nursery from giving newborn care. I don't know why he prevented us from getting our newborn experience at this hospital, but we had to travel to other hospitals to examine newborns—or secretly examined them at HPGH. We'd pull the curtains around the mothers' beds under the pretense of giving the mother privacy while we checked her and then we'd quickly check the baby also.

Not only was this rule ridiculous, but it put us in a bind. What would we do if we found something wrong with the baby? We weren't allowed to go into the nursery to read the baby's chart, so sometimes we wouldn't be sure whether the examining physician noticed the problem and informed the mother. Usually nothing was wrong with the baby and we could "sneak" our newborn experience and go our merry way.

But my luck went sour this particular day. As I examined the baby's hips, I found a hip click, which indicates that there was some hip displacement. The ball of the leg bone wasn't fitting in the socket of the hip bone properly. This abnormality usually is mild and requires only that the baby be swaddled in extra diapers, which serve as a binder to hold the ball in the socket until it decides to stay there on its own. Occasionally it requires surgery and a cast.

I wondered if the mother knew about the displacement. I asked her if the pediatrician had come to talk to her about the baby and she said she had.

"What did the doctor say?" I asked nonchalantly.

"She said everything was fine and we could go home tomorrow," the mother answered. Luckily she didn't pick up on my concern. I felt that the pediatrician should be the one to tell the mother of the problem.

I decided to see if the physician had noted the problem in the baby's chart. I left the mother snuggling her little one and went around to the nursery. I asked the nurse if any of the physicians were around so I could discuss a baby with them. There were none in the nursery so I walked around the postpartum unit to see if I could find one there. The floor was empty of doctors.

I ventured back to the nursery, and no one was at the nurse's desk. I quickly found the baby's chart and saw that the hips were checked off as normal. I decided to write in the baby's chart that I had noticed the dislocation. Maybe then a pediatrician would see it and follow up on my finding.

Feeling satisfied that I did all that I could do, I went to the nurse-midwifery office to rest my weary bones. Fifteen minutes later I got a call from the ever-so-hard-to-find-fifteen-minutes-ago pediatrician.

"You have no business going in the nursery! Nurse-midwives aren't allowed to set foot in the nursery!" she screamed into the phone. "You are not to touch the babies! And, you may not write in the chart!"

I let her scream it out. When she wore out, I explained my position. I spoke slowly and quietly. Finally she agreed to check the baby over again and discuss her findings with the mother.

The problem here was not that the physician was unconcerned about the baby but that we were both subject to a ridiculous rule that might have led to a lifelong deformity in this newborn.

One day I got a letter from the Washington, D.C. midwifery legislation committee that ultimately changed my life. Essentially, the letter informed D.C. midwives of the status of two bills that were up for vote by the D.C. Council. The first bill, being fought vehemently by the Washington, D.C. Medical Association, would give nurse-midwives and other nonphysician health care professionals admission and discharge privileges at D.C. hospitals. As stipulated in the bill, if a hospital deems a certain professional a competent member of his/her field, that hospital can then grant that professional hospital privileges even though he/she is not a doctor. Conceivably then, nurse-midwives, the experts of normal pregnancies, could admit a laboring patient, care for her, deliver her baby and discharge her without the supervision of a physician. Obstetricians, the experts of pathology in pregnancy, would care for those pregnancies that have or develop complications. And once midwives entered the marketplace, physicians would have to compete with them for business, lowering the cost of maternity health care. Today, this bill that passed in the early 1980's is law and it galvanized me into political action.

In answer to the nurse-midwifery bill, the D.C. Medical Association drafted their own nurse-midwifery licensing bill, which, among other things, stated that nurse-midwives would be allowed to deliver babies only in a hospital (eliminating birthing centers, a strong low-cost option to the traditional hospital setting). The bill also stated nurse-midwifery students can only be trained and supervised in the clinical area by physicians. The physicians lost this battle.

I delivered some babies at a hospital on the Eastern Shore of Virginia where there is a busy nurse-midwifery practice. The nurse-midwives in this practice deliver only indigent women. The students travel there frequently to get experience because of the high volume of deliveries.

One of the deliveries I attended was a woman who was having her second baby after a very normal first labor. We came on shift when the woman was fully dilated and ready to push her baby out. Betty, the head midwife in the practice, let her push for only a half hour and then called in the doctor to help "get the baby out." The scene that followed was so bizarre that I felt like leaving.

We were in the labor room. The doctor had one hand in the woman's vagina trying to turn the baby's head and his other arm was on her abdomen, pushing the baby out from above. Betty was helping him and commanding me to hold the mother's head to her chest. All the while, everyone was screaming, "Push! Push!" This was truly a forceps delivery without the forceps.

Suddenly the baby's birth was imminent, so everyone started screaming, "Don't push! Don't push," while we rushed the mother to the delivery room, scrubbed our hands, moved her to the delivery table, strapped her in and set up to deliver the baby. Finally, we were ready to deliver the baby and he plopped out into my hands.

After the placenta was born, the doctor ordered me to explore the uterus. This involves putting one's hand into the uterine cavity to get out anything that might be left behind, like blood clots or placental fragments. It is done only if the attendant checks the placenta and suspects it of being incomplete. It shouldn't be done routinely because it is extremely painful, it isn't necessary if the placenta is found to be intact, it can introduce infection into the uterus and it can traumatize the uterine muscle.

Because I was working under the supervision of a physician, I had to follow his orders. I apologized to the mother as I performed the procedure and I left the delivery with a heavy heart, not only because I hurt a mother who just had a baby, but also because Betty, a nurse-midwife, condoned the routine practice of this procedure.

Another delivery I attended at this hospital was for a woman who was having her first baby. After a few hours Betty came in, did a vaginal exam, decided the mother was seven to eight centimeters dilated and left. She returned a few hours later to check her, said she was the same, broke her bag of waters and told me to give the mother some Demerol for pain. The mother had never asked for medication.

After Betty left, I decided to give the patient a choice. I explained what I knew about the medication, and she and her boyfriend decided not to use the Demerol.

However, when Betty returned and I informed her that the mother had decided not to take the medication, she told the mother that her labor was going to get much worse and she should take it while she could. The patient gave in immediately. Betty taught me yet another lesson on the tremendous difference among midwives.

Betty had been a missionary in Pakistan and she trained to be a midwife there. Her midwifery training was very different from ours. We are taught to give people choices, support them, educate them, and promote the unity of their families. In Pakistan, Betty was in the middle of a sea of humanity cut off from the more sophisticated countries of the world. Health care was virtually nonexistent. Betty traveled long treacherous miles on horseback and in makeshift vehicles to secluded villages where she worked day and night to salvage mothers and babies weakened by disease, starvation, and hopelessness.

Once in the United States, Betty's practice remained to deliver the indigent. She worked with the poor who are neglected by the rest of society and most health care professionals. She delivers the babies of the women she sees in a clinic, and she has no personal relationship with them. She cannot afford to be sensitive to the needs and wants of these individuals. She has dedicated herself to literally saving her patients' lives. It was important for me to understand the differences between us. Betty frequently was all that stood between those mothers and hopelessness, despondency, and neglect. I could not compare our differences—only learn to respect them.

After I returned from the Eastern Shore, I started my clinical practice at a clinic for pregnant adolescents deep in inner city D.C. The nurse-midwives worked in a special program called "Community of Caring." It's a great health care program for pregnant teens where prenatal care is given by the nurse-midwives in coordination with social workers, nutritionists, counselors and doctors all under one roof. The pregnant young women receive a lot of attention and teaching during their pregnancies. The nurse-midwives do home visits before the delivery, so we know more about the patient's environment.

The philosophy behind "Community of Caring" is that the woman is a multifaceted person who needs to be educated on how to take care of herself and her baby to be successful in life. The more care provided, the healthier the mother and baby will be. The healthier the mother and baby, the more powerful they are to take control of their lives and turn failure into success. Our statistics boasted far lower infant mortality and higher birthweight rates than the rest of the city, and any other inner city in the United States.

I started this clinical with trepidation because I had always heard that teenagers were difficult to work with. But as time went by, I found out this wasn't true. In fact, they seemed to appreciate any attention they could get. I learned that as long as I was respectful as I gave information, they soaked everything up and tried hard to follow our advice.

As students, we had to choose a patient and follow her through her entire course of pregnancy from her prenatal to postpartum periods. I think I chose one of the "hardest-to-handle" teenagers for my case management study.

Margaret had hints of being receptive to care, but her heart already was a large void. She had been drained of all of her young life by an abusive situation in her home, and she no longer knew how to respond to care. It took her a long time to trust that someone was caring for her because she was suspicious of all overtures of kindness.

Toward the middle of her pregnancy I went to her house. The neighborhoods these teens lived in were so terrible that we were supposed to go on these visits in the afternoon to avoid the risk of being there at dusk. I visited her house one beautiful sunny morning.

Margaret had dressed up and she was wearing large hoop earrings. Her hair was fixed and she was wearing a dimestore engagement ring that she said her boyfriend had given her.

She introduced me to her aunt, and in the back room were some young men watching TV. She said they were her uncles. They didn't look up to acknowledge me as we walked through the room. In the bedroom she shared with her aunt, I checked Margaret's abdomen and listened to the baby's heartbeat. I let her listen too. We talked about preparing her room for the baby, and she showed me some clothes that her friends had given her. We talked about her baby-sitting arrangements. She said her aunt would be taking care of the baby. She was going to try to stay in school. I continually stressed to her how important that was. I detected a faint smile on her lips as she rolled her eyes at my often-repeated advice.

I tried to find out more about her boyfriend, but she was vague in her answers. If he existed at all, I couldn't tell whether he was the father of her baby. Listening to some of what she said, I began to suspect that one of her "uncles" was involved.

When Margaret went into labor, she couldn't deal with the stress. She became totally dependent and somewhat infantile. She even resorted to sucking her thumb.

When I arrived at the hospital, the doctor had already examined her and was sending her home, claiming she wasn't ready. Margaret was panic-stricken. She started crying when she saw me and soon afterward became hysterical, vomiting all over the waiting room floor. I took her back to a room and checked her again. There was no progress.

I wanted to keep her in the hospital, give her a sleeping pill and start an IV. That way she could sleep and get some fluids. Maybe then, some of her panic would subside. The doctor disagreed. She didn't want Margaret to take up an extra bed. We ended up sending her home in a taxi at 1:00 A.M. I felt awful sending her home, but I had no choice. The doctor didn't want to keep her and because only the doctor could officially admit a patient, we had to follow the doctor's orders.

At 4:00 A.M., Margaret returned. She was mentally bouncing off the walls. I kept her in the admitting office and tried to calm her down, but I couldn't. Finally, the only way I got through to her was to be stern. I told her that I wasn't having this baby for her and she had to take responsibility for her labor. I added that it didn't look like I was helping her at all, so I was going to leave if she didn't calm down. It worked like magic. She started relaxing with her contractions and, as long as I was around, worked beautifully. By 5:30 A.M. she was in good active labor and the doctor agreed to admit her, but Margaret's delivery was not easy.

We got her settled in the labor room. I moved slowly because I didn't want to upset her. As we walked through the hallways we stopped and breathed rhythmically together through her contractions. By 6:30 A.M. she was in her labor bed. I put on the external fetal monitor and after about fifteen minutes started seeing the baby's heartbeat go down. I changed her position and gave her oxygen, but the heartbeat got progressively worse. I called the attending physician. She agreed that things looked bad, but she said that she had to call in her chief resident before she could do a cesarean.

She left the room to call him. Officially the chief resident should always be in the hospital, on call for emergencies. She couldn't find him. He wasn't in the hospital. She tried to reach him at home but no one answered. It took her an hour to locate him to get permission to do the cesarean. Meanwhile, Margaret's baby's heartbeat was continuing to look ominous. I kept her on oxygen and continued to encourage her to breathe through her contractions. I was getting scared.

I joined Margaret in her labor breathing. I forced myself to relax. "Slow down, breathe deeply. Breathe in and out. Slowly," I kept repeating to her and secretly to myself.

I reasoned that if I could keep Margaret calm, less adrenaline would go through her system, and her deep breathing in her relaxed state would increase the amount of oxygen going to her baby.

The baby's heartbeat continued to look bad. Its slow ticking and decelerations with the contractions reminded me of a time bomb. Would it just go off? Or, would it die out gradually? The stark room seemed to echo the sound. After I prepped her for the cesarean, all I could do was wait.

The room was still except for the ticking of the heartbeat. I rubbed her back, her legs and her feet. She was very still.

I kept my voice low. "Slowly, slowly, breathe deeply," I whispered in her ear.

Suddenly, an hour later, the chief resident burst into the room with the other resident trailing behind, and Margaret received a cesarean eleven hours after she went into labor. The worst part of this story is that now her troubles truly began.

Margaret stayed on the postpartum unit for five days. She created havoc, or should I say she responded aggressively to the treatment she was given.

Her already restricted ability to establish rapport with people had fallen to the wayside. She threw her food trays against the walls, dropped banana peels in the hallway, refused to clean up her cigarette butts that she deviously planted on the floor beside her bed. Psychiatrists were called in. They concluded she was angry and promised they would return in the afternoon to start counseling. They never showed up again.

I believed that Margaret's problem was terror mixed with the poor treatment she received at the hospital. She sensed the nurses' hostility and responded without restraint or remorse.

I visited Margaret at home a few weeks after she brought her baby home. She had moved to another shabby apartment complex. I didn't know what to expect when I knocked on her door. Her "aunt" answered, but Margaret referred to her as her "grandmother" this time. Her "grandmother" showed me where to sit and went back to her soap opera. Margaret's baby was sleeping peacefully in his infant chair on the dining room table. He was beautiful. He looked healthy, and he had on new pajamas. Margaret's eyes sparkled. I sat with her and we talked for a while. As I prepared to leave the chair I was sitting on broke as I pushed it to the table. Margaret walked me to the door, and I hugged her good-bye. I hope she stays happy. I hope that she stays healthy. I hope she and her baby have a good life.

One of my last few deliveries at HPGH was one I will always remember because it was so beautiful. Tanya was an eighteen-year-old black girl whom I treated prenatally at Miller Place clinic. Her pregnancy was progressing without any complications when at her thirty-eight-week visit she sprung a surprise on me. She announced that her last menstrual period was in fact a month earlier than she had originally told us and she hadn't had intercourse at all the month in which we thought she conceived because her boyfriend had not been in town. This news put her thirty-eight-week pregnancy at forty-two weeks, two weeks overdue.

Because all other physical signs indicted that she was thirty-eight weeks, we speculated that there must be another reason why she suddenly changed her due date. Was it to protect the real father? Did she want to implicate another man? To be on the safe side, we sent her to the hospital for a nonstress test. With an electronic fetal monitor we listened to the baby's heartbeat. If the heartbeat elevates with each movement the baby makes, we can deduce that the baby is doing well. The nonstress test is often done with pregnancies that go past forty-two weeks.

After Tanya's announcement about the change in her due date, she and her mother started to become anxious. They both arrived at her next prenatal visit demanding to know why the baby hadn't been born yet. We handled them with explanations and some mildly confrontational questioning about the change in the date of her last menstrual period. Tanya avoided our confrontations by resorting to calling us instead of coming to the office. She would hang up quickly after receiving answers to her questions.

Then Tanya and her mother started to appear at the hospital admitting office with numerous false labors. Her mother was always nearby, nervously clinging to anything that was said. It became a standing joke that we were going to have to medicate Tanya's mother during Tanya's labor.

Finally her labor actually began, and I was glad it happened on my shift. Tanya arrived at the hospital at 10:00 A.M. Her mother was with her. Her contractions were very mild and her cervix was about two centimeters dilated. Her bag of waters was intact.

Teri was the instructor with me. We decided to send Tanya home because we knew that the sooner she was admitted to the hospital, the more interventions would be performed during her labor. We sent Tanya home with a repetition of the instructions that we had worked on during her prenatal care: danger signs and signs of labor. Her mother panicked at the thought of going home but, surprisingly, Tanya led her out of the hospital with confidence.

They returned about an hour later, complaining that Tanya's contractions were getting stronger and closer together. Her cervix hadn't changed. I gave them the choice to either go home again or walk around the hospital. Tanya wanted to go home, but her mother wanted to stay. We came to a compromise: I wouldn't ask the doctor to admit them but they could walk around the halls.

Before I let them out of my sight however, I gave her mother a lecture. Her babies had been born while she had general anesthesia, and she thought that was the only way women could have babies. Because she had never experienced the births of her own children, she wasn't the support she was supposed to be. She had carried the fear of childbirth throughout her life. I told Tanya's mother that I understood what she was feeling, but that now she was here to support her daughter. She had to stop acting fearful and be positive toward Tanya's labor and birth. I told her that I felt that her anxiety was causing Tanya to get anxious and that is not what giving support is all about. She assured me that she understood.

Teri and I left them to walk around in the hospital. About a half hour later, Tanya's mother called me to say they were going home. She felt a lot better and the contractions hadn't changed.

At about 2:45 P.M., we received a call that Tanya's waters broke and they were coming in to the hospital. We met them at the admissions office. Tanya's mother was in a state of panic again. Tanya's contractions were more intense and she was becoming anxious also. Her mother insisted that we give her an epidural. I put her off. First we had to get her admitted and that would take some time. Tanya received a bit of coaching from us and she worked with her contractions beautifully. I sent her mother to the lunchroom to grab some food while I went through the long admissions process. I had to repeat a history and physical, do the necessary admission paperwork of filling in endless forms, take blood work and a urine sample, start an IV and consult with the doctor.

Finally, Tanya was ready to go to labor and delivery. She started to feel the urge to push and her mother suddenly decided that she didn't want to go with her into the delivery room. I remember Tanya screaming at her mother, "What kind of mother are you that you would leave me at a time like this?"

Her mother never turned around as she walked away toward the waiting room. We wheeled Tanya into the delivery room. As we prepared her for delivery (getting her on the table, washing her perineum with betadine and draping her) we continued to coach her through her pushing. Tanya became totally involved in the process. Pushing required all of her energy and she became absorbed with the effort. Although I had to prepare my sterile table, I couldn't take my eyes off of her as she worked. I was fascinated by the birth. It demanded my total consciousness.

Tanya was purposeful. She listened to all of our instructions. I saw her mature into a woman in a few moments. She put all of her strength into delivering her baby. As the head was born, I told her to pant so that it would be born gently. Even though this is very difficult to do, she performed beautifully. The baby was born slowly and gracefully. Tanya's hands instinctively went out to bring her child to her breast.

When everything was over, we brought Tanya's mother back to the recovery room. She held the baby and all of her earlier fears melted into pride. She was proud of her daughter who had given birth in a way she thought was impossible. And she was proud of her first grandchild. Her eyes glowed with joy as she held him, and Tanya looked on with maternal pride. I left all three of them together to bond.

I was so happy for Tanya. Her work during labor was successful and her sense of achievement at having done it herself gave her the confidence she needed to hold, feed and love her baby. She was proud of herself and being the boisterous, talkative teenager that she was, I wasn't surprised when she later came to one of our prenatal classes with her baby to talk to the other pregnant teenagers. She told them how wonderful her labor was, how beautiful her baby was and not to worry because, when the time came for them to have their babies, they could make it good just like she did.

"Just stay with your midwife," she told them. "She'll help you through!"

Just as a stone thrown in a river makes ripples that spread to the surrounding water, the midwife who helps a woman labor successfully spreads her message through one woman to all the women around her. Just think, many stones could alter the river's current.

The last few months of midwifery school were hard because there were problems at home. My mother was truly incapacitated from her Parkinson's disease and couldn't even move. One day she called and asked me to come home from the clinic. I found her sitting in a chair with Ahren playing nicely nearby. She could hardly breathe. Her head, neck, back and abdomen hurt. She had taken her medications so something else had to be wrong.

I took her to a neurologist who put her in the hospital, but she refused all treatments because she didn't trust him. She wanted to come home. When I returned to pick her up at the hospital, she was lying in bed, rigid from lack of medication. I couldn't figure out why she fell apart so quickly or why she was paranoid and confused.

On the way home, the truth came out. If there was anything that upset my mother, it was soap operas. Once she started complaining about her hospital roommate watching the soap operas, I understood what had happened. My mother had a long standing hatred for hospitals and this, combined with her disorientation and her roommate's soap operas, was all she could bear. She had snapped.

By the time we got home, she was a little more calm, but she still was disoriented. By the next day, after I worked out a treatment schedule with her doctor, she was slightly better. But she was in no condition to take care of Ahren anymore. At times she was so incapacitated that Eric and I had to spoon-feed her. I bathed her and got her dressed every morning. Anneke read to her as she lay rigid on her bed. When she could talk, she complained because the doctor had cut her medication dosage in half. She believed that she needed twice the amount that they had prescribed. She was a pharmacist and no one could convince her that she was wrong. According to this doctor, she had been overdosing on her medications for a very long time. According to my mother, the doctor was working against her. She tried everything she could to get her medications back into her own hands. I refused to let her take them over because I believed that she was overdosing also. It was a difficult battle. On one hand, I hated to see my mother not have a choice over her own destiny. On the other hand, I started to see that this half dosage was working well.

I called my father in Holland. He quickly flew over and helped in her care. Over the days we saw her getting better and better, although she would still have occasional crises where she was totally incapacitated. My father nursed her well and took over her medication regime. I decided to step back and let them fend for themselves. My mother had turned quite passive and did everything my father said. This was good in one way but sad in another. She had always handled him with spunk and a good sense of humor, always managing to get her way. But now she merely echoed his thoughts and obeyed his commands. Luckily, because my father is a good person and her best friend, his commands were in her best interest. He made her eat well, take walks, get dressed in the morning and take a nap during the day. Yes, he was taking excellent care of her, but I still hated to watch her do everything he told her to do. It just didn't seem right.

They left for Holland three weeks later. I hated to see them go. What an odd mixture of emotions I had when I waved goodbye to them at the airport. My mother was passively waving goodbye, following my father onto the plane, which would take her far away from the people for whom she lived: myself and my children.

During the three weeks that my parents spent with me, I had time to reflect on their influence on me. Now that I had found my calling as a midwife, I wondered how that came about.

I'm sure midwifery was the furthest thing from my father's scientific mind. We never talked about feelings at home. Warmth and security were provided as a matter of course, but talking about it was just too corny. But even though the words "I love you" were never said, my father was always there for me.

I remember when I was little, waking my father up in the middle of the night for a glass of water. I really wanted to sleep with my parents at night. I was deathly afraid of the dark, and that was the only place I felt secure. I would see him at my bedroom door in his white boxer shorts. He brought me my water and sat next to me while I drank it. I'd drink the whole cup and then tell him I was feeling sick. This was his signal. He'd pick up my pillow and I'd follow him to bed. He never said a word to me the entire time. I just pattered behind him down the hall and snuggled into the middle of the bed. I didn't do this every night because I knew I would wear out my welcome. I strategically planned these night-time visits for about twice a week.

Throughout the years there were many times when my father came through and supported me, particularly when I was down. I wonder if this is where my patience to sit with laboring women comes from. I sit with them for hours without expecting them to perform. I just keep telling them that what will happen, will happen. Just be patient.

My mother was the dominant parent. She was the one who took on the major parenting roles. She lived with me, laughed with me, fought with me and without either of us knowing it, influenced me to be the stubborn person that I am. When I was a small child, she was home with me. A housewife, a mother. That's all I thought she was. I assumed that she would always love me and that she lived for myself and my siblings.

As I got older, I saw her branch out and develop her theories that I now know she was cooking up in the kitchen along with our dinners. My mother was different. Most of my teen life, her difference embarrassed me. Why wasn't she like my friends' mothers? Why did she have to intervene when the principal spontaneously decided to dismiss school early because we had finished our testing? My peers glared at me as she towered over the principal while he announced into the loud speaker that no more students were allowed to go home.

"You can't let these children go out into the streets unsupervised!" she admonished him. "Their parents don't even know they're out of school!"

I watched my mother fight with doctors about my health. I was sickly and they wanted to hospitalize me a few times but she wouldn't let them. At one time she was willing to have our house quarantined by the public health department because she wanted to keep me home when I had viral hepatitis and the doctor wanted to isolate me in the hospital.

After I had my own children, I began to understand my mother. As a mother myself, I was stubborn, and not willing to let anyone take care of them.

I watched my own mother with my children. I saw how much she loved them and how she was ready to dedicate her life all over again to their well-being. She never tired of giving love. She never tired of giving to me. In a way, a mother is a midwife as she supports her children through each new phase of their lives. Just as a midwife, she gives them the support they need, the energy they need and the possibilities they need. But then, just as a midwife, she has to let go to let them go the course they have chosen. The support, the energy, the possibility . . . my mother gave those to me. Now, I give them to other women.

This support is difficult to give in a hospital setting where you have to care for many patients at one time. You just do not have the time to give the patient support during labor so you use technology and medication to help yourself out. A woman who is strapped to her bed by an electronic fetal monitor, and who cannot walk because she has an epidural is less demanding and allows you to meet all of your other demands like hospital paperwork, other physicians and other patients.

An unmedicated woman, on the other hand, draws all those around her into her labor: She demands that they support her and labor with her. Helping a laboring woman is hard physical and emotional work. More often than not I am exhausted after being with a woman in labor. Clearly the "medicated" management is easier for the provider. That's why the majority of women receive pain medication. It's a support substitute. And, you can look like you're caring for someone by manipulating all of the medication and technology. Medication and technology are your crutches and the patients are so impressed by your ability to manipulate the machines that they think you are caring for them.

8

I GRADUATED from the Georgetown School of Nursing on December 10, 1983 with a Master of Science in Nurse-Midwifery. I knew I should have been elated on my graduation day, but my happiness was marred by the empty seat in the audience where my mother should have been sitting. She had worked as hard for this as I had, but she wasn't able share it with me. I resolved on that day that I would never let her leave my thoughts. During the rough times that would surely follow I would draw on her image to see me through.

Immediately, the job offers came rolling in. I interviewed at the University of South Carolina in Charleston. It was beautiful and the job security was great, but when they offered me a position on their faculty, I knew I couldn't do it. Two more job offers rolled in.

I cornered Eric on a bright and sunny New Year's Day. "We have to make a commitment now," I said.

Eric thought the situation through. He knew what I wanted. I was committed to providing safe choices for women for childbirth and I wanted to start an independent home birth service. He knew what he wanted. He was tired of working in the public schools. He wanted to develop his music career and he also needed more time every day to manage his psoriasis. Because we were committed to avoiding day care for our children, he decided that home employment was the option for him. Yes, even though it was a huge financial risk, we both knew that we needed to do what we both wanted now. And because the job market looked good for nurse-midwives, I could always get a job if things didn't work out.

So it was settled. On January 1, 1984 my service was born.

Designing my own business was exciting and overwhelming. As I created objectives, protocols and budget plans, I was glad that I took those graduate administrative courses. On paper, things shaped up quickly and nicely, but my insecurities raged within me. I could only hope our decision was right. Eric resigned his job effective at the end of the school year. His salary would continue through August, but by September the burden of supporting the family was going to fall on me.

My insecurities seemed not to impress Eric. In June he put his energies into finding an inexpensive place to live. We focused on the Shenandoah Valley in Virginia. I loved its beauty and peacefulness with the Blue Ridge Mountains protecting it on all sides. It gave me a sense of security. Eric's eyes were on the low cost of housing. We found a quaint little house in Winchester and with the help of my parents, we bought it.

After developing the administrative side of my business, I had to find some doctors who would back me up, or, as stated in Virginia law, "supervise" me. In Virginia, a nurse-midwife must work under the supervision of a physician. "Supervision" is a poorly defined term, but it means that the physician has to be available to collaborate with the nurse-midwife or the patient.

This was the beginning of a long history in my service of the perils of working under the supervision of physicians. Of course, because some pregnancies and deliveries can become complicated, the American College of Nurse-Midwives (ACNM) recommends that we work in consultation and collaboration with physicians, but not under their supervision. Certified nurse-midwives are the experts of normal pregnancy, and we are licensed to practice our profession in accordance with standards outlined by the ACNM.

We are registered nurses who have been educated in a program that is accredited by the ACNM. The ACNM is recognized by the U.S. Department of Education as an approved educational accreditation agency. At the successful completion of an accredited nurse-midwifery education program, we have to pass ACNM's national certification exam. The ACNM is a member of the National Commission for Health Certifying Agencies, which sets standards for organizations that certify health professionals for clinical practice. After passing our national exam, we are certified and eligible for licensure in all of the fifty states. To maintain our certification, we must continue to take courses in our field throughout our careers.

Obviously, our certification is not a learner's permit where we can't practice unless a physician is sitting next to us to supervise our every move. However, we must be able to practice in situations where we can consult and collaborate with a physician in the event of a complication (just like a general practitioner consults with a specialist when he detects a health problem that is beyond his scope of practice.) As far as liability, we are accountable and responsible for our own management decisions and the physician should only be held liable for his direct decision making and participation in client management (again, this would be the same as the general practitioner/specialist arrangement).

The American College of Obstetricians and Gynecologists (ACOG) advises its members to maintain their supervisory status through "close chart review and close contact." But, what does that really mean? Maybe it means that the patient must see both the midwife and the physician each month and the midwife must bring her charts to the physician to review. Maybe it means that the midwife must notify the physician every time she sees the patient or make regular "check in" calls to him. Terms like "close chart review" or "close contact" are nebulous terms and up for individual interpretation.

One thing we know for sure is that "close contact" between midwife and physician has never been shown to increase the well-being of our patients, and never has a physician's "close chart review" of a midwife's chart increased the quality of the midwife's care. We also know that this kind of position taken by ACOG is unrealistic because it increases the cost of health care. The patient would essentially have to foot the bill for this duplicity in care. And a physician would have to be awfully good-hearted to put up with constant interruptions, day and night, by a midwife clamoring for his approval of her every action.

The bottom line is that midwives and obstetricians are in economic competition for the same client. By continuing to demand that we work under their supervision, physicians can keep us from practicing independently and therefore they can keep us from threatening their existence. Because I'm legally dependent on my competitor for my existence, my position is a frail one indeed. (If a small hotel had to ask Holiday Inn's permission to operate in the same area, what do you think their answer would be?)

Obviously, this was the one issue that I should have had a lot of doubts about, but because I so desperately wanted this service to succeed, I refused to pay attention to my misgivings. I just knew there was a physician out there who would agree with me. Of course, this was my biggest problem. Because I was covering a large rural area, I needed to find as many supervising physicians as I possibly could. Even though I was lucky in those first years, the task of finding them was formidable.

The first physician, Dr. Moore, practiced in Timberville, a small town in the Shenandoah Valley. I heard from the traditional midwives that he supported them and was excited at the news that a CNM was coming to the area. I went out to see him in early February.

The drive out to his office was beautiful. The Shenandoah Valley is truly one of the most scenic areas in the nation. There were patches of snow dotting the mountain ranges and the bright crisp day added to my sense of well-being. I knew that I would love living out here. I knew that I would find peace nestled in those old mountains.

His office was in the hospital, which was in the middle of town. The nurse greeted me pleasantly and led me to his office. Dr. Moore entered and we shook hands. I made a note of his limp handshake.

He didn't look like a happy man. His face was puffy and he was over-weight. I knew from the traditional midwives that his wife, also an obstetrician and once his business partner, had just left him. He was in the process of getting a divorce.

He didn't want to know much about me. He wanted to tell me about the other midwives in the area.

"I've been supporting the lay midwives in this area for a long time," he began. "I don't know much about them though. I just know that when they get in trouble, they come in and I just fix things up."

I listened silently. I knew what was coming: a tirade about the traditional midwives. I wanted to steer clear of this. I vowed to myself earlier never to discuss the traditional midwives with doctors. It seemed unnecessary and unfruitful.

I changed the subject.

"How long have you been here?" I asked.

"A long time and I can't do this by myself. I'm trying to find another doctor to come here with me, but I can't seem to attract anyone to this area."

I sensed burn out.

"It must be difficult to be on call twenty-four hours a day and never have a break," I said sympathetically.

I leaned forward in my chair.

"Here are my protocols," I said. "These are the rules by which I practice and I'd appreciate it if you'd look these over and see if you agree with them."

He started leafing through the protocols.

I watched him.

He continued to talk as he went through the cumbersome forty-page document. I could tell by his expression that he was impressed.

"Where are you planning on living?" he asked.

"I'll find a central location in the valley so I can serve the Shenandoah and Northern Virginia areas," I answered.

"You'll find the cost of living to your liking out here, I suppose," he mused.

"I'm sure I will compared to the Washington, D.C. area."

"Well," he said, placing my protocols on his desk. "I'd like to see your patients once a trimester."

I explained that I had access to a laboratory and would do all of the prenatal lab work.

"Good," he said. "Send 'em to me after the first visit."

He pointed to my protocols. "I like these," he grunted. He signed them and handed them back to me.

He rose from his desk. "Good luck to you and it'll be a pleasure working with you."

The visit seemed easy but I felt unsure inside. I didn't trust him. The way he talked about the traditional midwives bothered me. And, because he made no effort to find out about my practice philosophies, I wondered how long it would be before he talked about me the same way. I knew I needed to find more supervising physicians in case one of them backed out on me.

The next physician I met with was Dr. Peterson, a general practitioner in a town west of Clarksburg. I had heard about him from the home birth midwives in the D.C. area. They said he was very supportive and even did some home births himself.

It was late in the evening when I drove to his office in a small quaint town west of Clarksburg. I drove through a small main street lined with colonial mansions on both sides. The setting sun cast a soft glow on their balconies. His office was in a small rancher right before the town's only intersection.

Inside I found myself among a few patients still waiting to see the doctor. I told the receptionist I was there and settled down to leaf through an old *Good Housekeeping* magazine. While I looked through a few more out-of-date magazines, my attention strayed to my surroundings.

How plain everything was. There was nothing ornate or pretentious about this waiting room. Interior decorating definitely was not on this man's mind. I liked that because I knew that when an office is fancy, the patients paid for it. An older woman in street clothes took me back to his office. I noticed that none of his employees were wearing uniforms. I liked that too. They were regular people.

She showed me into his office and invited me to sit down. After I declined a cup of coffee, she left, cheerfully assuring me that he would be right in.

"Actually," she said rolling her eyes with a smile on her face, "don't count on it. He gets to chatting with his patients and we never see him again!"

I settled back and quietly surveyed the room. The most accurate way to describe his office was "disorderly." The furniture was old and imposing. The brown paneled walls had diplomas and certificates cluttering them. His desk had a glass covering that was hidden beneath piles of this and that. Only he could know where everything was.

I liked this man before I saw him. He was a country doctor and one whom I suspected lived by the Hippocratic oath.

Dr. Peterson walked in with a relaxed gait, as if he had all the time in the world. He was an older man, quite handsome and healthy looking.

"Good," I thought to myself. We nurse-midwives joke that because back-up physicians are hard to find, we like it when they are healthy so they will be around for a long time.

He took my hand in a gentle but firm handshake. He invited me to sit down and walked around to his desk. His manner put me at ease right away. I leaned back in my chair. He joked around a little bit and welcomed me to the area.

"I'm glad you're here," he laughed. "I'm getting too old to go out to people's homes and stay there all night. I love it too much to give home births up entirely, but I sure could use someone else out here."

"You think I'll get enough business?" I asked. My insecurities showed through my careful professional manner.

He smiled at me. His blue eyes were sympathetic and kind.

"You'll be fine. People will be knocking down your door soon. Hang in there." He signed my protocols. "Anything you need, just give me a call."

I knew he had a few more patients so I rose to go even though I wanted to stay. This man was refreshing. He had no hidden agendas. He was just an uncomplicated doctor, one who gave the best care to whomever came into his office. I knew that very little threatened his ego. He was solid.

I walked out of his office into the cold night air. I felt exhilarated. The bright starry night reflected the clarity of my purpose. I was going to make it. I just knew I would.

The third physician I met with, Dr. Mendel, was from the same area as Dr. Peterson. He was also a general practitioner and seemed very supportive of home birth. He was a more intense man however, and I felt uncomfortable with him. He was young and still trying to prove himself in the medical community. He referred to the other doctors, how they were quick to intervene in the delivery process and how they were giving him a hard time. He used to do home births but he didn't anymore because of the pressure he had received from his peers. We met for longer than I liked and I politely took my leave as soon as I could.

My misgivings about Dr. Mendel were correct. A few months later I had the opportunity to test his support. Elaine, one of my clients, started bleeding in the third month of her pregnancy. After I checked her, I called Dr. Mendel. Elaine had chosen him as her back up physician because he was her family doctor. He enthusiastically agreed.

When I called him, he answered the phone immediately. I told him Elaine's problem. He said he'd meet us at his office and take a look at her there and then take her to the hospital if needed.

I tried to soothe Elaine on the way to his office. This was her third pregnancy and had not been planned. She was upset that it had occurred, but now that it was threatened, she wanted it more than ever. I clasped her hand. Her blond hair was covering her face as she cried. She was a gentle woman and already I liked her even though we barely knew each other. I sensed that our professional relationship would blossom into a personal one.

We pulled into Dr. Mendel's parking lot. He met us as we got out of the car.

"I've decided I don't want to back you up," he said.

We looked at him in surprise. It was not even a week earlier that he had told Elaine that he would be her back-up physician. Now she was bleeding in his parking lot and he was backing out.

"Why?" I managed to utter in my surprise.

"I don't feel like it would be good for my practice at this time," he answered. "Just go to the emergency room and use the doctor on call for walk-ins, and don't use my name because I don't want them to think I had anything to do with this."

He turned and walked to his car, not bothering to show concern for Elaine or even to say goodbye to her. We stood in his parking lot and helplessly watched him drive away.

We called Dr. Peterson, and he met us in the emergency room. He ordered an ultrasound and determined that the pregnancy was normal. He consoled Elaine. It was probably just slight bleeding from her cervix but nothing to worry about.

"Just take it easy for a few days," he instructed.

He turned to me. "Call me if this happens again."

Meanwhile, my other interactions with physicians were not going in the right direction. I called one doctor in the Washington, D.C. area who had been referred to me by one of my classmates. He sounded enthusiastic about me being in the area when I called him. He was used to working with midwives and looked forward to meeting me.

"It's really important that we have trained professionals doing home births," he said.

My hopes were up. "Wow, this is easier than I thought!" I said to myself. I made an appointment to see him.

Because he was near one of my clients, she decided to use him as her back-up physician. I told him of her plans and he said, "Send her in!" Unfortunately, my client's appointment to see him came the day before mine. He called me up after her appointment and sounded entirely different.

"What do you think I am?" he screamed into the phone. "Do you think

I'm just some second rate provider that your patients can use when they get
in trouble?"

He just kept yelling into the phone. I had no time to talk. I was offended
by the foul language he used, so I hung up. My patient told me later that
he told her at her visit that he would not work with me.

With his rejection came a new lesson that is still difficult for me to overcome. It was painful for me to have this man yell at me and I took it personally. How could someone be so pleasant and then be so awful? I hardened
a little bit. "Don't trust the doctors," I said to myself. "And, if possible, stay
away from them."

In the late winter and early spring I started to get calls from clients. Because
I didn't have an office, I made all home visits. It was interesting finding out
about how people lived. This is the most fun and colorful part of my service:
my clients, their homes, their families. You learn so much by being in people's
homes. Besides all the dry stuff you ask on the forms, you learn their loves,
their talents, their tastes and their desires. You watch them be wives, mothers,
daughters and friends. It is only in the home that you see someone at their
best and at their worst. And, because I believe women's labors reflect their
lives and their individuality, it's important to get a feel from the woman's
whole being, not just her uterus. I was really taking care of people where
they needed it . . . in their homes. And, because my clients had access to my
home number, I was also taking care of them when they needed me.

I never knew what I would find when I knocked on my clients' doors for
the first time. They came from a wide variety of settings. In that first year I
had a chiropractor and his wife. I had two families in which the fathers were
carpenters. One of my clients had just finished EST training. One was in
the business of selling vitamins, and I got a sales pitch from her at each of
my visits. Another client was a teenager, living with her boyfriend and their
one-year-old daughter.

Elaine, another one of my patients, pulled out dozens of bottles of herbs
and glandular extracts when I asked her the routine question about whether
she was taking supplements. I smiled when I filled up the back page of her
chart with the names of some of the supplements, such as pancreatic enzyme
from a horse's pancreas. My chiropractor client taught me various massage
techniques. The fascinating world of holistic health was opening up to me.
I came back from my prenatal visits with a head full of ideas and questions
and a heart full of joy. I was doing what I wanted to do.

During the spring I did a number of community publicity drives to promote midwifery and my service in the area. I felt that people needed to know
that midwifery was a viable alternative to a traditional medical practice.

I got the midwifery film *Daughters of Time* from ACNM and went to nursing schools, childbirth educators' meetings and public meetings at various community libraries. I used these events to emphasize the miserable infant mortality rates in our country and how the promotion of midwifery would increase the access to prenatal care and therefore decrease these high rates. Moreover, I made the point that the lack of prenatal care made women unhealthy and more vulnerable to the interventions that made birth so dangerous.

I was always worried that no one would show up at these events. My stomach was tied up in knots as I drove out to the different communities. I was so convinced that women needed my service that I wouldn't have been able to bear it if no one showed up. Of course not as many people showed up as I would have liked, but I enjoyed doing these events and I still have friends today that I met then.

Also in the spring I was invited to give a speech to the Larsonburg Junior Women's Club at their next banquet. I consented, seeing the importance of penetrating this conservative community.

I wrote a speech about the childbirth reform movement, childbirth education and midwives. I emphasized a mother's right to choose the type of care she wants. I practiced my speech over and over again so that it would go smoothly because I'm only too aware of my nervousness in front of a group of people.

I was successful in keeping calm during my drive to Larsonburg. Two-and-a-half hours of open highway is very hypnotic. When I arrived at the hotel where the banquet was held, I sneaked into the bathroom to change out of my scrubby jeans. All of a sudden there was an amazing transformation! A road-weary nurse-midwife with tee-shirt and jeans became a sophisticated professional with business suit and pumps . . . all within the confines of a hotel bathroom. As muzak piped through the vent, I put on my make-up and went over the crucial parts of my speech in front of the full-length mirror. I emerged fresh, articulate and appropriately dressed, ready to take on the world. But, as I entered the banquet room, my new-found confidence started to crumble. In fact, panic set in. What was I doing here? What do I do now?

I spotted the past president of the Junior Women's Club. She came up to me and quickly ushered me to my seat. Hurried introductions were made between myself and my table mates.

I felt queasy. The table was so formal. I desperately searched these women's faces for some signs of warmth and understanding but they basically ignored me and talked among themselves.

The next half hour was spent struggling with my silverware and the fried chicken. Another surge of panic set in. I made a mental note for the future to turn down any requests for speeches at banquets where fried chicken was being served. It definitely requires preliminary preparation in etiquette.

When the time came to give my speech, I numbly followed my hostess to the front of the room. She introduced me and I stepped to the podium to begin. The words sputtered at first but became more fluent as my resolve grew stronger. (This always happens to me when I talk about midwifery.)

Applause came slowly afterwards and when it died down the questions started. I sensed hostility about midwifery and my home birth practice. I desperately searched the audience for a sympathetic smiling face. I saw none.

"C'mon Juliana, keep standing. You can get through this," I coaxed myself.

The first comment went something like this: "I don't see why anyone would want to have their baby at home. I went to the hospital, did my Lamaze breathing, and made it through just fine. I don't think the mother has the right to choose home birth because she's placing her helpless baby at an unnecessary risk."

My answer: "That's your opinion and even though statistics don't support you, you have every right to your opinion. However, people have opinions other than yours and they too have a right to all of the options. Our job is to make their choices safe ones."

The next question: "Where do you get your statistics?"

She quieted after I quoted three sources.

A woman behind her asked, "Are you trained in endotracheal intubation?" (Endotracheal intubation is a particular resuscitation technique where a tube is placed down someone's trachea through which oxygen is pumped into the lungs.)

"Yes," I answered.

Both women looked at each other dubiously.

"You mean," the woman continued, "that all nurses are trained in endotracheal intubation?"

"Endotracheal intubation is not routinely taught to nurses on the undergraduate level," I answered. "However, I have a master's degree in nurse-midwifery and endotracheal intubation is a required skill in the nurse-midwifery curriculum."

A woman stood up in the center of the room.

"I sense you are being attacked," she stated. "But, let me tell these ladies about my birth! I was in the hospital with my first child with a ruptured bag of waters and labor didn't start for three hours. My doctor got tired of looking at me, so he used pitocin to start labor. I went out of control during my contractions so they put on an epidural. Of course, since I was numb from the waist down, he did a forceps delivery. My bladder was traumatized, so I had to have a urinary catheter. I stayed in the hospital for more than a week. I had my next two children naturally because I wouldn't let anyone near me. I'd jump at the chance of working with a nurse-midwife."

I didn't have time to respond. A string of questions shot at me from all directions.

"How does the traditional medical system accept you?"

"Do you do a lot of education in your prenatal care?"

"Do you stay with the mother during labor?"

"Do you encourage and help with breast-feeding?"

There was a lot of buzzing around the room. The president beat her gavel on the table to calm the room down.

As they quieted, she stated, "One more question."

A woman timidly raised her hand. "What's your phone number?" she asked.

That same spring I helped to start the Virginia Chapter of the American College of Nurse Midwives. Eric had always told me that if I wanted to be a nurse-midwife, a major part of my job would be political.

"Juliana, your profession will be eliminated by the medical community if you don't do something new," he warned. "You're a threat to their existence and they won't tolerate it for long."

"No, that won't happen to us," I thought naively. "People will just understand that we're right and the medical community will never succeed in getting rid of us."

The upcoming political events that occurred in the state taught me that Eric was right.

At the end of March our chapter had its first meeting. I looked forward to it, not only because I saw it as a way for Virginia midwives to unite and protect themselves, but also because I wanted to renew some of my contacts with other midwives in Virginia. Five midwives came to the meeting held at my friends' home in the mountains west of Charlottesville. It was a cold, crisp spring day. The wood stove was burning and we all gathered around its warmth. Three of us were nursing our babies and toddlers were playing with toys at our feet. At times our conversation could barely be heard over the chatter of the children and the rattling of their toys.

Even though there were only five of us, our backgrounds were sufficiently varied to create an exciting tone. Three of us were friends as nurses in Charlottesville and all of us were now midwives. We all had home birth practices. The fourth was a midwife from northern Virginia who worked in a health maintenance organization, and she had been one of my preceptors during my gynecology clinical at school. The fifth midwife was an older woman who worked for a physician in southwest Virginia. She was elected as our first chapter chairperson. She believed strongly that midwives should work closely with physicians within the traditional hospital setting. However, she also believed that there was a fine line between this type of midwifery practice and the type the physician wanted: midwife as servant to physician.

I agreed with her. We needed to work together with physicians yet remain legally autonomous. I knew that if physicians had their way, we only would be allowed to work in their offices under their supervision, doing their work and making their money. We would lose all of our rights, and eventually our identity. We all agreed that we needed to do everything to prevent us from crossing that fine line.

I looked over the women around the stove. We were all mothers, we were all midwives. Two demanding full-time jobs. It would seem we couldn't stand a chance against the medical community who had their meetings in the Bahamas. I remembered reading an article about how doctors became so powerful over midwives and effectively eliminated them. It wasn't because their care was superior to midwifery care, it was because doctors were men who could leave their wives at home while they traveled to professional meetings. At these meetings they formed cohesive groups that could influence legislators to create laws protecting the medical profession through the elimination, or severe restriction, of other kinds of health care professionals.

Meanwhile the midwives had to stay home to tend to their families. Unfortunately, midwives didn't have the opportunity to unite in the same way as doctors and fight for themselves politically. And we're far behind in wealth and prestige, which is what frequently buys the legislators' votes.

But there was power in our camaraderie. It wasn't money power or political power. It was a far deeper power. It was the sense that we were the guardians of the most precious people on earth: mothers and children. It was our calling to protect them and ourselves.

I watched our hostess, Julie. She had replaced Laurie, the midwife who delivered Ahren, as the local nurse-midwife doing home births in the Charlottesville area. Laurie had long since stopped practicing because of the pressures of the medical community. I watched Julie with her one-year-old son, a severely retarded baby. I sensed a lot of strain behind her soft eyes. My heart went out to her. She had had her share of harassment from the medical community, and now, because of the work involved in taking care of her son, I knew she would be gone soon. Judy was replacing Julie. Charlottesville had already seen two midwives come and go, and I wondered how long Judy would last. She was pregnant, due to deliver in a few months. Midwifery requires a determination to fight anyone who stands in your way. That's difficult when you have your own newborn baby in your arms. I hoped that Judy would have that unknown ingredient that it takes to be successful in this field.

Our first meeting was productive and we all left with our individual organizational tasks to perform. There were by-laws and standard rules of practice to create. We had to recruit more members, set up committees and nominate the officers. By May, everything was completed and I began my term as vice-chairperson of the Virginia Chapter.

Our chapter was barely born before it had to address problems that came up in the state. The first was an effort by physicians to restrict nurse practitioner practice. (Nurse-midwives are legally nurse practitioners in Virginia.) Our struggle with this issue taught us the valuable lesson that the assaults on our practice were not necessarily direct but were more likely to be tied in with other political occurrences.

In the early 1980s the federal government redesigned the Medicaid requirements that each state had to meet to receive federal money for providing Medicaid services. One requirement was that each state was required to include nurse-midwives as independent Medicaid providers. That meant that nurse-midwives could bill Medicaid for their services without a physician's co-signature. Each state had until 1984 to implement the protocols necessary to allow us to become independent Medicaid providers. Of course, the federal government wanted more nurse-midwives as Medicaid providers. They had long ago researched nurse-midwifery statistics and found that we provided safe, cost-effective care. And, wherever nurse-midwives practiced, the infant mortality rate dropped. As long ago as 1932, the Metropolitan Life Insurance Company of New York estimated that if nurse-midwifery services were adopted nationwide, the perinatal (the time from twenty-eight weeks gestation to twenty-eight days old infant) mortality rates of the time would have been reduced by 60,000 per year. In light of the dismal showing the United States was making internationally in infant mortality rates (the nation's rates were the eighteenth highest of twenty civilized nations), nurse midwives were a good idea.

The medical society of Virginia didn't like these Medicaid requirements, not because they were interested in providing care to Medicaid women, but because it further legitimized our practice and opened the door for private insurance companies to follow the government's direction. Once insurance companies reimbursed midwives directly, more people would be attracted to using a midwife and we would get a chance in the health care marketplace.

The medical society of Virginia tried another tactic. They adopted a "Maternal/Child Clinical Pregnancy Risk Evaluation," which placed women in different risk categories. There were many factors for evaluating women such as medical history, pregnancy history, family history, and socioeconomic status. Each factor was given a number based on its importance. A score above twenty would make the patient too risky for a nurse practitioner to care for.

There is value in a risk evaluation system but, if carried too far, it can become restrictive. For example, the Maternal/Child Clinical Pregnancy Risk Evaluation rated a past history of a bladder infection as a ten. It also rated a family history of diabetes as ten. So, basically, if I had a bladder infection in my past and my grandfather had diabetes, I couldn't have a nurse-midwife deliver my baby. And, because it was very easy to reach a score above twenty, this tool would rule out most low-income women. So, if the state adopted these guidelines, most midwives, whether they were Medicaid providers or not, wouldn't be able to work.

Meanwhile, we caught wind of another, more direct attack. The Virginia Obstetrical and Gynecological Society felt that nurse-midwives in Virginia were not being adequately supervised. In other words, nurse-midwife practices were growing too independent. So in 1983, they adopted the following resolution:

> Resolved: That the Virginia State Board of Medicine should license nurse mid-wives to practice only under the direct supervision of a qualified Obstetrician-Gynecologist who has full active staff privileges in a J.C.A.H. approved hospital in the same community that the mid-wife practices. Should such an association terminate, the license of the mid-wife should be temporarily suspended until another association with a qualified Obstetrician-Gynecologist is established.

How were we to practice under that resolution? First of all, some physicians who supervise us are not obstetricians, but family practice and general physicians. By requiring that only obstetricians supervise us, the resolution severely limited the pool of physicians who would work with us. Second, what does "community" mean and who sets the boundaries? Was it meant as a social or geographical term? Finally, the society's statement gave doctors far too much power. If a physician wakes up one morning and decides he doesn't want to supervise us, our license gets suspended. What a set up for extinction.

The Virginia Obstetrical and Gynecological Society sent this resolution to the Joint Boards of Nursing and Medicine who actually regulates our practice. The Joint Boards knew that this statement would never be legally adopted because Governor Charles Robb, to decrease the administrative load of regulation and to increase the access to health care providers, was commanding all regulatory boards to trim their regulations and eliminate unnecessary restrictions of the practice of all health care professionals. But, under increased pressure from the wealthy and powerful obstetrical society, the Joint Boards finally adopted a statement that included a provision to ensure that the physician review all of a nurse-midwife's cases at least once a month.

This statement also was unacceptable. First of all, I would have to drive to two or three physicians' offices every month so that they could review and sign my charts. The patients would end up paying for this duplicity in care. And there has never been any evidence that this kind of monitoring of the midwife's care increases its quality. It only increases restrictions and decreases the access the public has to our care.

These events spurred our chapter of the ACNM into action. We focused on the administration's deregulatory efforts—they were good for all non-physician health care providers.

Our major debut was our speech to the Joint Boards. This was the first time our chapter was meeting our regulatory Board formally, face-to-face. We wanted to make a professional impression. We wanted to show that we were professionals who were here to stay. I worked for days preparing our speech. I designed it to go hand-in-hand with the governor's specific deregulatory directives. My point was to show that requiring us to get our charts signed monthly was directly against these directives. The paper flowed smoothly because it was so obvious that this was an unnecessary restriction.

We debated for days on who should present the speech. We finally retained a lawyer to speak for us. I primed him on ACNM policies, nurse-midwifery standards of practice, anti-trust issues we faced and our statistics. Later, as I sat behind him when he presented my speech, I saw that his nonchalant posture, his untucked shirt and his loose tie made his poor attitude glaringly clear. For a moment I had the horrible thought that the future of our practice in the state rested on this joker. I promised myself that I would never do this again. If I had something to say, I would say it myself. From then on, I became the speaker for our group.

Luckily, we won our battle about the monthly chart signing and in the remainder of the year we had other victories as well. We got a nurse-midwife appointed to the Advisory Committee to the Joint Boards of Nursing and Medicine, and we helped develop and implement the rules for Medicaid reimbursement for midwives. The only goal we had that we didn't meet was to get a nurse-midwife appointed to the malpractice review board of the state to protect us in future liability issues. All in all, we felt pretty successful in 1984, but we realized there was a long hard road ahead.

In the summer of 1984 I attended my first home birth. The couple, Lucy and Michael, were living in Richmond. I'm still amazed that I agreed to do their delivery since they were so far away from my home. They called me though because the midwives in their area worked with a doctor who performed abortions which, as born-again Christians, Lucy and Michael opposed. I met with them three times before their baby was born.

Lucy went into labor one morning in early June. Her bag of waters broke at 2:30 A.M. and she had started mild contractions at 5:30 A.M. I decided to go ahead and go to their house so that I wouldn't have to rush later.

It was a beautiful drive, and when I arrived they were relaxing around the house. Both of them were cheery and excited about the impending delivery. Her contractions were coming every fifteen minutes and they were only about thirty seconds long. She smiled at me as I timed a few of them. I knew we had a long way to go.

I didn't do any vaginal exams because she had a broken bag of waters and I didn't want to expose her to infection. I encouraged them to go about their daily activities as normal and I listened to the baby's heartbeat and took her temperature throughout the day. (If her temperature rose, I would have to worry that she was starting an infection that would be dangerous for the baby.)

I spent the day reading some articles I had brought with me, and finishing some chapter paperwork. I even cleaned out my car. We took walks together and, while they napped, I got to know their dog, a crotchety old poodle who was soon to be replaced as the baby in the family.

All through the day they were visited by members of their church. I sat respectfully by as they prayed together. Everyone was so positive toward Lucy and gave her everything she needed from spiritual support to covered dishes. The minister even came by to offer his blessings to their baby and their home. I could see that her faith was the basis of her strength and her community of friends had taken it upon themselves to help her through. She was fortunate to be able to gather these people around her. This is one of the things home birth allows a mother to do, have a baby in her world, her domain, where she is boss. And, she can invite anyone she wants. In fact, if I wanted to have someone come with me, I'd have to get her permission. How many women in hospitals feel free to tell a strange doctor or nurse to leave the room? Not many, because it's not their domain. That's the art of home birth: to preserve the mother's sense of control over her environment, because when there is a sense of control, there is no fear. I loved the thought that she could go on about her daily business under my watchful, unobtrusive eye.

As the day wore on, Lucy settled into her labor. Her contractions were steadily getting longer, stronger and closer. I went over to visit some friends from college who lived in the area. I was wrapping up quite an enjoyable day. After dinner, as I was reminiscing about good old times with my friends, the phone rang. It was Lucy. Her contractions were getting harder now. They were every three to four minutes and sixty seconds long. She had one while we were talking on the phone and she stopped talking to me so she could concentrate on it.

"Hmmmm," I thought to myself, "This sounds promising!" I hugged my friends goodbye. They wished me luck.

I arrived to find her in her bedroom with Michael and two of her close friends. One of them was my birth assistant. They were gently massaging her and praying. I quietly sat on the floor next to her and coached her through the contractions. Her face was blushed, her eyes were bright. Her baby's heartbeat was doing well and her temperature was normal. Here was a healthy woman in labor. It was truly a beautiful sight to behold.

The time flew by. It was already past midnight. She was starting to feel like she needed to bear down. In fact, with a few contractions she was bearing down involuntarily. I did my first vaginal exam. She was completely dilated and ready to push her baby out. We put her on a stool at the foot of her bed. I laid out sheets to protect the floor. I let her urge to push build up on its own. I've always felt that the gentle bearing down a mother does of her own volition is far more effective than the forced pushing we make women do in hospitals. I kept her sitting on the stool, sometimes on the toilet. I've always felt that the more upright the mother is, the more effective her labor is because we have the help of our best friend, gravity. And there's nothing that enhances one's sense of control more than having both feet on the ground.

Her labor was getting very intense; her urge to push was very strong. I could tell the baby was moving down. Her friends were chanting prayers into her ears. They started speaking in "different tongues." It seemed like the mother and her friends were in a trance together. I watched with fascination. Her husband was sitting behind her supporting her back. I monitored the baby and the mother's blood pressure. I wiped her forehead and occasionally interrupted their chanting to give her some instructions. She would open her eyes, smile at me and nod her head. She was very peaceful.

Lucy was pushing harder and harder. I started to see the baby's head. More and more of it showed with every push. Finally, after two hours of hard work and pushing, the baby was ready to be born. I wanted her to push the head out slowly to avoid any tearing of her perineum.

"Try to blow while you get the urge to push," I said to her.

It was hard for her to do. I blew with her to keep her focused. Everyone joined in. We were all so involved, it was as if we were all having the baby together.

"Blow, blow, blow," I repeated.

The baby's head appeared slowly, first its scalp and forehead, then eyebrows, then eyes and nose. The mouth popped through, then the chin. The head was out! I wiped away the mucus that was being pushed out of the mouth. We waited for the next contraction. (I always call this moment the longest in the history of humankind.)

It came. The baby's head turned to face the mother's right side. That was the signal that the rest of the baby was ready to be born. She slid out into my hands.

"A girl!" I heard Michael say. "It's a girl!"

The baby sputtered and cried.

"Praise God. Thank you Lord. Praise the Lord." I heard these exclamations around me as I dried her off and lifted her to Lucy's arms.

Lucy clasped her to her breast. Everyone was crying. Michael and Lucy were cooing to her. They untangled her blanket and checked her out. I sat back and watched. I couldn't hold back my own tears. I'll never tire of watching this miracle.

While I watched them, I busied myself with the tasks I had to perform after the birth. I kept an eye on Lucy's bleeding as I waited for the placenta to come out. I let it come when it was ready. There's no need to pull it out; this is a dangerous practice that can lead to hemorrhage.

I checked Lucy's perineum for a tear, found a small one and sewed it up. Then I got her settled into bed and let her enjoy her baby. She breast-fed right away. I examined the baby and went to sleep. They would make an appointment with their pediatrician the next day.

In the morning, I tiptoed into the room to check on them. The whole family was in bed. Michael was sound asleep and Lucy was lying with her baby nestled in her arms. I went over to her side and quietly gave each a final check before I left them in the hands of my birth assistant. Michael slept through it all.

The ride home was long but joyful. I turned up the radio and sang old rock-n-roll songs. I thoroughly enjoyed myself. When I went back two days later, the carpet cleaners were there cleaning the bedroom rug. Apparently one of the plastic sheets had a hole in it and it had leaked over their white carpet. To this day, whenever I see carpet in someone's bedroom, I remember the strange looks those cleaners gave me as they were cleaning the carpet. I also check all plastic sheets before I put them down.

A few days later, my other patient who was due in June went into labor. This was their first baby too. Marianne was a sweet and positive woman. Her husband, Brian, was a chiropractor. He was dark and very quiet. I never knew what he was thinking or whether he agreed with me. He was very involved in alternative health care. In fact, I didn't know how deeply involved he was until the birth when we clashed over how I managed a complication.

Prenatally, I always go over emergencies and complications of birth with my clients. We talk about what we will do in the unlikely event that they might occur. From this discussion I know where my clients stand and how they will react in an emergency situation.

Marianne's labor was long and hard. I was at their house for a total of 24 hours. The baby was posterior, its back facing Marianne's back, so she had a lot of back pain. My birth assistant was trained in massage therapy, so we were lucky to have her share in the back rubbing job. We all took turns at it.

That first day her contractions were mild and fifteen to twenty minutes apart. We fixed dinner together and watched TV. I got a massage from my birth assistant. We all went to bed early. My birth assistant and I slept in the living room on sleeping bags.

In the early morning Marianne's contractions started to get harder. Her back started hurting more. We walked together and then I sat her on the toilet for what seemed like an eternity. She took many baths. Her labor progressed slowly but surely. I bonded well with her. We laughed together and solved the ills of the world between contractions.

The day turned into night. We greeted midnight together. Marianne seemed to be the most comfortable on her hands and knees in bed. That's the way the baby was born two hours later. I'm glad she was in that position because the infant's shoulders were wide and difficult to deliver. Because she was on her hands and knees (Gaskin Maneuver), I could deliver the baby's bottom shoulder first even though it's the baby's shoulder facing the mother's front that's usually delivered first.

Because the baby's shoulders were so difficult to deliver, he was limp at birth. The delivery took longer than normal and it was hard on him. I suctioned him quickly and thoroughly as my birth assistant brought over the oxygen tank. He responded well to the suctioning and with much grimacing and sputtering, he let out a solid yell before we could give him the oxygen. His body pinked up and by one minute of age he was squalling. I put him on Marianne's belly.

I covered them both up. Now to check on Marianne's uterus. I quickly felt Marianne's abdomen to see how well her uterus was contracting. It wasn't. I massaged it to encourage it to contract. She started bleeding heavily and the placenta still had not yet come out. I encouraged her to push it out and because she was unsuccessful, I concluded that it must have been partially attached. Emergency! The uterus can't contract with the placenta still partially attached and she was hemorrhaging from the place in the uterus where the other part of the placenta had detached. The only thing I could do was put my hand into her uterus and gently scrape the remaining part of the placenta loose.

I warned her that this was going to be a painful procedure. She saw the urgency in my eyes as I was talking to her. She nodded her head and assured me that she would work with me. I was grateful that we had developed such a trusting relationship. It meant the world to both of us at that moment.

She performed her rhythmic breathing technique while I starting working the placenta loose gently but firmly as I had learned in school. It detached readily. I pulled it out while I held her uterus in place. My birth assistant was ready with my emergency medications for hemorrhage. I administered those immediately. Her bleeding went to a normal level.

I got the baby to nurse so that his suckling would also stimulate her uterus to contract. He attached himself to her nipple like an old pro. When I was sure her blood pressure was stable and her bleeding was fine, I busied myself with straightening up. Finally, I went out to the living room to gather my wits.

I sat on the couch and stared at the wall. I felt my hands start to shake. My nerves were taut, like a stretched rubber band. I needed a quiet place to let them loosen up and relax. I closed my eyes and started breathing deeply and regularly. I concentrated on relaxing every muscle in my body.

"C'mon, Juliana," I kept saying to myself, "Keep it together. Everything's under control now."

I heard some quiet footsteps come into the room.

I kept my eyes closed. I knew it was the husband, Brian.

He stopped next to me. I looked at him.

"Did you really have to give her those shots?" he asked me in a very irritated tone of voice.

I looked at him in amazement. My nerves and muscles snapped back. I knew he was involved in alternative therapies but I thought he understood that in emergencies, I was going to use my medications. I sat bolt upright. My face flushed with anger. As far as I was concerned, I had handled a disastrous situation quite well. I felt my eyes flashing.

Very quietly and very slowly I said to him, "Look, we had two emergencies in that room, a very difficult delivery and a partial separation of the placenta with hemorrhage. Your wife is in there nursing your baby. Those emergency techniques and medications made that possible. Now, if I were you, I'd be in that room basking in the glory that a healthy mother and baby can bring to a family."

He looked at me intensely with those dark eyes of his. I looked back at him steadily, daring him to say a word. He turned away and walked back into the room.

I leaned back on the couch. A new level of tension in my body made it impossible to relax. My birth assistant came out to sit with me. She rubbed my back. I calmed down and set about caring for the mother and baby.

I stayed many hours to make sure they were fine. I called my back-up physician, told him what happened and warned him of the possibility of the need for antibiotics because I put my hand inside of her uterus. Even though we use sterile technique, there's always the possibility of infection.

Marianne was wonderful as always. She got up to clean herself and, with our help, did quite a good job. The baby was beautiful and nursed frequently before he went into a peaceful sleep. I left them with the baby sleeping at her breast.

Brian was friendly to me during those hours, but I couldn't easily forgive him for his criticism and his suspicious attitude. I experienced for the first time the rejection of one way of health care, when one is oriented toward another way. Just as medical doctors reject a lot of alternative therapies, people who practice alternative therapies reject medicine as it is practiced today. Both sides are wrong. It's important to use the most effective therapy for your client no matter its origin. To me, that's the beauty of nurse-midwifery. Because we can practice in the hospital or at home, our dedication to preserving individualism invites many to receive the best of both worlds while still staying in control of their destiny.

The rest of the year passed relatively peacefully. I found a literary agent to promote a children's story I had written in 1980. It was published in *Ms.* magazine in September.

I worked in a temporary position as a nurse-midwife for the faculty at Georgetown throughout the summer, delivered babies at HPGH, and moved into our new house in the fall.

Our home was great for my business. Its location was convenient to major highways, and there was a cute sunroom upstairs that I used as my office. I proudly fixed it up with my desk (a Woolworth special that my father bought when I was three), a mattress on the floor and my bookshelf for books and lab equipment.

Over the years my office got more sophisticated. I put in an actual bed, lab table and microscope but I still stubbornly hold to the idea that I didn't want it to look like a doctor's office where sick people go. I loved its homey feeling. I had a colorful quilt on the bed, mobiles and pretty shades on the nine windows. There were children's drawings on the walls alongside my diplomas, and at the door I had a big bulletin board with snapshots of many of the babies I've delivered. There was a big basket of toys for children and a loveseat so my clients could sit comfortably with their partners.

My family and I went to Holland for three weeks in August to visit my parents. I was so happy to see my mother again and she was in her glory having us there. We all had a great time but when it came time to leave, my heart made that old familiar plunge. I felt it coming for days. It's like a pit in my stomach and the only way to relieve it is to cry desperately. But, I fought my tears as I waved goodbye to my mother. She was at her bedroom window, waving to us, waving goodbye to her children, her reason for living. Finally, when I was safe in my airplane seat, I let my tears flow unchecked while Anneke and Eric held my hands.

After we settled in our new home, I enrolled Anneke in the third grade at the local public school and Ahren in the local Montessori school. Eric got a job working part-time as a speech therapist for two agencies. The job was great because he picked Ahren up at noon and they were both home for lunch.

I met with a physician in northern Virginia who signed my protocols and still continues to be one of my most trusted back-up physicians. Over the years, he has gone through some harassment from his peers but still is steadfast in his support of me. I thank him and admire him.

The rest of my deliveries that year were beautiful and uncomplicated. One was with a family having their fourth child. Their Great Dane (the largest Great Dane I ever saw) greeted me at the gate every time I came for a prenatal visit. He loved to jump up and put his paws on my shoulders. Often the children would lasso him and save me. Their mother delivered a sweet little baby girl one sunny warm morning. The other children and the grandmother were present for the delivery. By then, the kids were all pretty used to me so they were singing and chattering quite freely. The oldest girl, a six-year-old, was very serious as she helped me get the room ready for the delivery. It was my first delivery where siblings were present, and I will never forget the wonderful sounds of astonishment they made when they saw their little sister being born. I feel it's a privilege for them and their new little baby.

I delivered a baby boy to a couple deep in the country. They had no running water, and it was scary going to the outhouse in the middle of the night. The moon was bright, the air was crisp and the animals were restless. An old goat's bell tinkled as she followed me across the field. I was sort of glad she came with me; I wasn't so alone then. As I was in the outhouse, my mind flashed to all the things I'd done to become a midwife. I fought through two more college degrees and now was fighting in Richmond to retain my status. I'd spoken to executives at their board meetings, to hospital administrators and at legislative hearings. I'd learned how to play the part of executive businesswoman. If they all could only see me now, in an outhouse in the middle of the night with a goat patiently waiting to walk me back to the house. When the baby was born in the wee morning hours, I looked up to see my friend, the goat and three of her buddies staring in the window.

A baby boy was born to my client who was left bleeding in the parking lot by Dr. Mendel. It was a rainy day and we sat in her kitchen for hours while she rocked in her rocking chair. Her roof started leaking and we watched the water trail down the stone chimney. She had invited her friends at the local rescue squad to the birth so, as the father and I delivered the baby together, the chief of the rescue squad, knowing that I wanted the birth time, kept calling out the time exactly to the second.

"Twelve thirty five and fifty seconds, twelve thirty six and two seconds, twelve thirty six and ten seconds." His voice could barely contain his excitement even though he was trying to sound official. Finally the baby's cries and the exclamations in the room drowned him out.

I learn many valuable lessons at each of the births I attend. One of my first lessons was that many people who called for my services did not necessarily subscribe to the philosophy of the home birth movement. I learned quickly that just as not all midwives are alike, not all people who choose home birth are alike. Not all of the people who called wanted the privacy, the dignity and the "naturalness" that come with having a baby at home. A lot of people called me because they didn't have insurance and they couldn't afford the doctor and hospital. Some midwives balk at doing home births with people who don't have the "home birth" philosophy, but I decided immediately that I was going to provide the best care that I could provide for everyone who called. And that's exactly what everyone got. Through 1984, I did all home visits, and spent many hours with my clients.

I got to know their families very well. Essentially, my job was to keep people safe as they made the best decisions for themselves.

One couple, Tina and Tom, delivered at the very end of the year. They lived in a quaintly renovated schoolhouse on an old southern plantation. Their house was beautifully designed with baskets, natural materials, sheepskins and dried flowers.

Tina's labor progressed beautifully with no problems. This was their first baby so her labor was quite long. We enjoyed the day together and late in the evening, we all went to bed to try to get some sleep. I went upstairs with my birth assistant while Tina and Tom went to bed downstairs. Their friends, a couple from out of state, slept on the living room floor next to the stairs.

In the middle of the night I had to go to the bathroom so I tiptoed down the stairs. Tina had a large blanket hanging beside the stairs. I thought it was a wall so I leaned against it to enable me to tiptoe lighter. Suddenly, I felt the blanket give way and I fell down the stairs right in the middle of the couple sleeping on the floor.

What a shock it was for them to find me in their bed. They screamed as they jerked awake. My birth assistant bolted down to help me. Tina jumped out of bed and came running into the living room.

"Are you all right?" she gasped as she fell to her knees beside us.

"I'm fine," I assured her. I was still sitting in between the couple.

We all burst into laughter.

Suddenly Tina's labor picked up and after a few hours of contractions, she delivered a beautiful baby boy. What a way to get someone to deliver.

Right before Christmas I delivered a little girl to a mother having her third baby. Carol's bag of waters broke first so I spent the day with her. She would have contractions for a few hours and then they would stop for a few hours. Normally, I wouldn't have spent the day there, but those few hours of labor were always intense enough to look like they might be close to producing a baby.

We had a fun day together. She worried that she couldn't go to her son's Christmas party at school. He had been looking forward to her coming for a few weeks and she knew he would be really disappointed. I thought about it for awhile. "Why not?" I thought to myself. I packed her into the car and we went to the Christmas party. Her son's eyes lit up when he saw her come into the room.

After the party we decided to go Christmas shopping. I had my stethoscope along and listened to the baby's heartbeat in the car. At the mall I bought a coat for Eric and Carol got some toys for her kids. We got home by late afternoon. She took a nap and woke up at dinner time with strong contractions. Their baby girl was born an hour later. The kids were excited that she came before they had to go to bed. I went home after that birth satisfied with a great delivery, and satisfied that I got some Christmas shopping done!

On New Year's Eve I reflected on my past year. It had been busy. I started my service, started the Virginia Chapter, and got my story published. I even set up a contract with a nursing school for students to observe my practice. I attended some great births and some hard ones.

Yes, it had been a good, productive year. My family was healthy. I was still mom and a midwife. And, I loved it.

9

MY FAMILY always teases me that I see everything in terms of pregnancy, labor and delivery. Indeed, we all have our frameworks within which we try to understand life and its cycles. In my framework, my first year out of school was the embryonic and fetal stage of my service. The second year was going to be the birth. I knew it was going to be a good one. I had taken such good care of it during the pregnancy.

I had so many plans for the year. My major one in the beginning of 1985 was to start a birthing center. By the mid-1980s, it had become apparent to more and more people that the maternity system in the United States was in deep trouble. The national infant mortality rate was higher than that in eighteen other countries and the price of having a baby was at least $3,000. Many women couldn't afford care and therefore were losing out on the valuable education that prenatal care provides. Complicating the issue was the shortage of providers, so that even if a woman could afford care, she was often unable to find someone who could give it.

The result of both situations was an increase in low birthweight babies whose likelihood of dying before their first year was high. And if they did survive, their likelihood of poor performance in schools was higher. The emotional, social and monetary costs of these babies was becoming incomprehensible and too much for our society to bear.

The rural states were being hit the hardest. Generally, low-income states attract few providers. The only solution these states had was to deregulate— to decrease the barriers against providers who weren't physicians and facilities that weren't hospitals. These states became perfect places for midwives to set up birth centers. West Virginia was one of these states.

Winchester is located about twelve minutes south of the West Virginia border. In one town, Charles Town, about twenty-five minutes from my home, there was a community of people who subscribed to alternative methods of health care and living styles. Whenever women in this community needed traditional medical care, they went to Dr. Wemsah, the only obstetrician in town. Before I arrived, he backed up midwives who traveled from the Washington, D.C. area to deliver their babies. When I met with women in this community, they told me about Dr. Wemsah. They respected him and attested to his loyalty to the welfare of mothers and babies.

I made an appointment to see Dr. Wemsah late in 1984. He was a small, energetic man from India who spoke quietly and quickly. He pointed out the pathetic situation of many of the women he saw in his office. They couldn't afford the basic necessities of life, much less their obstetric care, so he saw many of them for free. Here was a sensitive man who was truly concerned about the state of our society.

He also spoke of the medical system. His expression changed from worry to disgust as he told me of the unwillingness of many of the doctors and hospital administrators to address the problems.

So many impressions went through my mind. His attitude fluctuated between worry, anger and despair. Indeed, as he lifted his hands helplessly in response to discussing solutions, I saw the ingredients of burnout pervade this man. He was exhausted in his solo struggle of providing the best possible health care for the women of the community.

I recognized his feelings from my nursing days. Back then my soul had burned with frustration because I knew people weren't getting the care they needed; indeed, I'd actually seen many being neglected or abused. Since then I'd been searching in all directions to find a solution within the system. I hoped that somewhere, somehow, I could penetrate and make a lasting change that would improve the care women and babies received. But the health care system is an arrogant old monarch, firmly entrenched in preserving its own infallibility. Change comes reluctantly because change infers that the way things are currently being done is wrong and it requires someone to do something about it. But, even though many well-meaning individuals enter the system with high hopes of accomplishing something, too many of them end up—like Dr. Wemsah—exhausted and frustrated. I wasn't going to let that happen to me. I wasn't leaving the system because of burnout, I was leaving to transform it from the outside in.

As I sat across from this man, I realized that he was a precious gem that must be preserved. If change was going to come to this area, he would have to be the force behind it.

"Maybe," I thought, "maybe there's something we could do together."

A little bit of my idealistic self surfaced again. I started romanticizing.

Maybe we could start a birthing center! In a birthing center I could give prenatal care and do deliveries in a comfortable home close to the hospital. The facility would be simple so that its cost would be low, and safe so that low-risk women could deliver there. I could hire other midwives to work with me. Dr. Wemsah would be the consulting physician with the responsibility of delivering the higher risk women and the women we have to transfer from the birthing center. That way his work load would be significantly decreased because he wouldn't have to deliver all of the women in the area.

I excitedly told him my thoughts. He watched me intently as I spoke. He was quiet when I finished. I barely noticed his hesitation. I was suddenly so sure that this might be a great solution to two problems: the lack of care women receive and Dr. Wemsah's burnout.

"Your plan is a good one," Dr. Wemsah said. "Bring me an outline of it on paper and we will discuss it further."

I went home and told Eric. He agreed that we should look into this option and the next few months were dedicated to formulating this plan. We researched the area thoroughly: studied its past, present and projected demographics, physician to population ratios, infant mortality rates, and teen-age pregnancy rates. We contacted the state of West Virginia and started the procedures to open a not-for-profit corporation. We filled out the tedious forms to obtain state grants. I went to community events and city council meetings to meet people and glean as much information as possible about the area. Intermittently I would meet with Dr. Wemsah and describe our progress. He continued to encourage me. We even traveled together to a birthing center in Maryland to talk to the staff and tour the facility.

Finally, during one of our meetings, he told me that the medical staff at the hospital had gotten wind of my plans and was not very supportive. The general practitioners also delivered babies, although they stayed away from the low-income women. They, of course, recognized the potential competition a birthing center would impose. It was well known that women would travel great distances to deliver in a birthing center. They were popular, and would also attract higher income women.

"Of course," Dr. Wemsah warned me, "the hospital administrator is very influenced by the medical staff. Maybe you should go meet with him because I don't think we can do this without his support."

I had a sinking feeling that I was losing Dr. Wemsah. He had been talking to the medical staff and he was feeling their pressure. I drove home. I was thoroughly depressed. I should have seen it earlier, I should have listened to my suspicions. Dr. Wemsah wasn't ready yet. He was still feeling shackled by the system and not ready to break free.

A few weeks later I met with Mr. Daniels, the hospital administrator. He was a short stocky man who curtly invited me to sit down without shaking my hand. I saw immediately that if he wasn't on your side, he would be a formidable enemy.

"So," he said as he settled back in his chair behind his desk. "What can I do for you?"

I had rehearsed my presentation so that I would present my birthing center as a complement to the hospital rather than a competition. No such luck. He was determined to snuff this project out.

I felt that my presentation was complete. I covered all of my bases. I answered all of his questions. They were the typical ones and I prepared well for them. Then the conversation took a turn that I had not prepared for.

"Are all of the patients in this birthing center going to have natural child-birth?" he asked me.

"Yes," I answered. "No medications for pain will be given since they increase the incidence of complications for both the mother and infant."

"Are husbands going to be with their wives for delivery?" he asked.

"Of course we'll encourage family centered births," I answered.

He chuckled. "Well, even though we let husbands in with their wives for delivery here too, I don't think it's a good idea at all. I read a study that said that a lot of men became impotent after watching their wives deliver a baby." All I could do was stare at him. He curtly dismissed me.

Again I drove home depressed. I knew we were doomed. I called Dr. Wemsah right when I got home. Mr. Daniels had already called him. Our conversation was quick.

"I talked to Mr. Daniels today," I told him.

"Yes, he called me," he said. "He doesn't like it at all."

"I think I figured that out," I answered.

"Maybe we should wait a little while," he decided. "The time isn't right at this moment. I will continue to watch for the right time. I will call you then."

I hung up the phone. I couldn't believe it. It was over, just like that. In one breath. All of my work, all of my energy, all of my hopes. Gone. As usual, I went to Eric for consolation.

"Dr. Wemsah wasn't ready," he told me. "Your original intuition was right. But all of our work isn't gone. It's just put on the shelf to use another time. Everything always works out for the best."

I wondered what I would do without Eric.

Despite the disappointment I experienced with my birthing center, I plunged forward into my births. I had no choice; these babies were going to be born no matter what mood I was in. Shortly after New Year's Eve an early morning call woke me at 5:00 A.M.

Eric answered the phone. He was half asleep.

"Not much, Dave. What are you up to?" he said in response to the caller's question. "Let me give you over to Juliana."

I took the phone. Dave and Mona were having their first baby. Only a few days before, I had met Mona in the parking lot of a furniture store to do a prenatal visit. I was concerned about her baby's heartbeat. I thought I had detected an occasional irregularity. I called Dr. Peterson about it and he told me to check it again for awhile and if I still detected it, to send her in for more testing.

When I called Mona to arrange for this extra visit, we decided to meet at a furniture store that was close to her home and on my way to another one of my prenatal home visits. I figured that I could just put back the seat of my car and listen to the baby's heartbeat for about ten to fifteen minutes. Right after I pulled up to the parking lot I decided to check in with Eric. It was closing time for the furniture store but after I explained the situation to the owner, he let me in to use the phone. After I got off, the owner told me that in his country midwives were quite popular. His accent was familiar so I asked him where he was from. "Belgium," he answered.

We spoke Dutch together, and when Mona arrived he invited us in to do our prenatal visit in his store. We welcomed the warm alternative. I listened to the baby's heartbeat while Mona lay back on a stack of beautiful Belgian rugs.

Now, only a few days later, her bag of waters broke. Dave was excited when he talked to me on the phone. Mona hadn't started labor yet so we reviewed all of her instructions and danger signs on the phone. Because she was two-and-a-half weeks early, I requested that they see Dr. Peterson for a second opinion on the size of the baby. I had detected no irregularities in the heartbeat at the furniture store so I wasn't concerned about that.

They called me up after Dr. Peterson's visit to say he OK'd a home birth. The day wore on and we kept in contact by phone. I had them call me every two hours with an update. Her labor started in the early afternoon. As the contractions got closer, we stayed in contact more frequently. Finally, I went over to their home in the evening.

They were fixing the bed when I arrived. Mona had napped throughout the day so she was well rested. I fixed dinner for them, tomato soup and turkey sandwiches, and we watched "Dallas." My birth assistant arrived.

Late in the evening, Mona's contractions started getting quite intense. She paced around the room while we watched. She'd sit on the toilet frequently and Dave rubbed her back when she was on the bed. Everyone worked hard. We took turns helping Mona. Sometimes we rubbed Dave's back while he rubbed Mona's. We tried to encourage Dave to go take a nap but he didn't want to leave Mona for a moment. He finally fell asleep in the bed while it was our turn to rub Mona's back. The night moved into early morning. The clock ticked away. We walked and walked.

It's amazing how long it takes a baby to be born. As time passes slowly, labor gives one the opportunity to reflect on the process of birth. Each contraction comes and goes, never to return, but while it's there, it seizes the moment to shorten the uterine fibers so that the uterus gets smaller and smaller. As the uterus gets smaller, the baby is massaged down further and further into the pelvis. Sometimes you can see a mother's abdomen change shape and become almost pear-like as she walks. Finally, the uterus, getting more powerful as it decreases in size, pushes the baby out of its first cradle, the pelvis, through the vagina, the passageway to life, into the outside world. The mother, feeling more and more pressure, joins the uterus in its expulsive efforts. She bears down gently and involuntarily at first but then more forcefully and purposefully as the baby approaches birth.

In its natural environment, giving birth is like a musical masterpiece, building to its crescendo when the baby enters the world. Just as a symphony pulls its audience into its powerful rhythm, so does a laboring woman pull in her onlookers. All of those present at a birth must be in synch just as all of the instruments in an orchestra must be in synch. This synchronization helps the mother keep her power to create her own masterpiece. Often, in the wee morning hours, when her privacy is assured, her baby is born.

Mona's labor built up to the point where she started to feel the urge to bear down. Her cervix was completely dilated and I felt the baby's head low in the vagina. She squatted while she pushed during the contractions and walked during the break between them. She found it most comfortable to lean on the banister in her hallway while she pushed. It was there that she delivered.

As the baby approached delivery, my birth assistant and I moved all of my equipment into the hallway. We put plastic sheets under Mona as she leaned on the banister overlooking her living room one floor below. Dave was still behind her, supporting her hips. I encouraged her to push while I got under her to monitor the baby's heartbeat.

Finally, the head appeared. Dave was behind Mona, sitting on the floor. I was beneath her in the front. Together we had our hands around the baby's head, supporting it as we coaxed her to push the baby out slowly. A beautiful little boy was born into Dave's and my hands. I held the baby as Dave eased Mona back onto his lap. His arms were around her as they both welcomed the baby into their arms. My birth assistant covered all three of them with blankets to keep the baby warm with their body heat. We turned the lights low so the baby would open his eyes. In happy exhaustion, we sat back and through our tears watched this family fall in love with each other all over again.

Even though the births often exhausted me physically, they gave me the energy to keep up the increasingly heavy load that my business had become. It was taking up more and more of my time. There was so much to do, so many avenues to follow to ensure that my service would become a cornerstone in the community. I continued to meet with doctors and work out arrangements with nursing schools in the valley to be a guest lecturer and preceptor for nursing students.

By the time the nursing students started coming to my office to observe my care, my schedule had gotten fuller so I couldn't do all home visits with my clients. I had decided to do the first visit and the thirty-six week visit at my clients' homes while the rest of my prenatal visits would be in my office. Not only did the students attend my office hours but I also took them to home visits with me.

I enjoyed having the nursing students along. I felt that it was good for them to see this kind of care. Too often in nursing school, students are only exposed to the medical management of childbirth. While they were with me, I could expose them to a whole new concept of women's health care. I could show them that as a professional nurse-midwife, I could help women take care of themselves and deliver their babies in dignity and safety. I wanted to show them that this was real nursing care—teaching people to take control of their own health.

I wanted the nursing students to think about the possibilities for themselves as independent providers of nursing care. I wanted them to look at the system from the outside in and see that care can be provided in another way. I wanted to ignite the fire of curiosity in their minds and encourage them to wonder if the system was working in its present state. Finally, I wanted them to see me work within the framework of my home and family. Most of us are women and eventually most of us become mothers. The nursing profession is plagued by members leaving to stay home with their children and by childcare issues for those that stay in the workplace.

I like to encourage women to stay home and work out of their homes. Nurses who are mothers can become pediatric nurse practitioners, geriatric nurse practitioners and even obstetric-gynecological nurse practitioners and stay home, seeing their patients in their homes. It's discouraging to see motherhood being abandoned for careers. But, it's also discouraging to see careers abandoned for motherhood. Teaching people to take care of themselves within their own moral, social and personal orientations is the cornerstone of health care and is what motherhood and nursing are all about. The two careers can be combined and done in the home if the nurse and patient choose.

Occasionally, when a nursing student was with me on a home visit, I would get called for a birth. This is what happened one snowy evening. Renee called me with steady contractions. They sounded strong enough for me to come right over. When we arrived, they had slowed down significantly but because this was her second baby and she was four centimeters dilated, I decided to stay. Barbara, the nursing student, had no choice but to stay also.

Renee was a single woman who thought she was married to a man but found out that he was a bigamist. She left him early in her pregnancy and moved to an apartment above a store in a small town in the valley. She and her three-year-old daughter lived together in the cozy three rooms upstairs. Her parents came by frequently to help her.

Because Renee's labor slowed down, Barbara and I decided to go to the diner next door to eat dinner. By the time we came back, her contractions had picked up. We went back to her bedroom and sat on her bed. Barbara was starting to look a little pale. Her period had started and she had terrible cramps. She lay down on the rug. Renee got up and fixed her a hot water bottle. A little later Barbara really started getting sick. Sweat broke out on her brow. We fixed her tea and periodically Renee wiped her forehead with a washcloth. I had to smile at Renee. After all, she was the one in labor and she was taking care of the nursing student! I tried to take over the job.

"No, it's OK," Renee insisted. "This keeps my mind occupied."

I let her go on, wishing I had a picture of her squatting beside the ailing nursing student.

Eventually, Barbara fell asleep and Renee settled down to labor. Her sister-in-law came to watch her daughter. We sent them to bed. Renee lay down on her bed and I lay down next to her. We dozed between contractions. Periodically she'd wake me with the contraction. I'd listen to the baby's heartbeat and lie back down.

Suddenly she jumped up. The bag of waters broke. She felt the baby coming. I got up, put on my gloves and caught the baby in my hands. Renee was semi-reclining in the bed. I handed the baby to her and she nursed immediately. They settled back into her bed and I pulled the cover back over both of them. Barbara stayed sound asleep on the rug beside the bed, waking only slightly to look confusedly at her surroundings and go to sleep again.

A few days later I delivered another baby to a Mennonite family on a dairy farm deep in the valley. I enjoyed working with the Mennonites. Words cannot accurately describe these people. They are so straightforward and uncomplicated. Their faith in God is direct and simple. It is their way of life. There is no proselytizing and I had the sense that they accepted everyone from everywhere. We are all equal in their eyes.

This couple called me during the previous fall and this was their second baby and first home birth. I'll never forget my first visit with them. It was in the early evening when I drove down the valley to their home, tucked away in the farm country that was mostly inhabited by Mennonites. Occasionally, I'd pass a black horse-drawn carriage with a fluorescent diamond on the back to warn approaching vehicles of its presence. I turned into their driveway, passing the milk storage tank and barn before I pulled up to the house.

My patient, Elvira, greeted me at the front door and showed me to the living room. She was a slight woman, with her hair wrapped tightly into a bun inside of her small white cap. Her gray dress was high-collared. She sat down in a straight-backed chair across from me. She apologized that her husband was still in the fields rounding up the cattle.

My first home visit with my clients was divided into three parts: the history, an explanation about my service and the physical exam. That night the history seemed long and painstaking. There are many intimate questions that need to be asked, and she shyly answered them in a voice that I had to struggle to hear. Actually, I started feeling shy myself. I'd never asked such intimate questions of a Mennonite woman who was so deeply religious. The room seemed to get quieter and quieter. I almost felt like apologizing to her.

Finally, we finished. Now I had to explain my service. Jerry, her husband, hadn't arrived yet so she murmured quietly that she would call him in. I nodded and bent my head to finish up some writing that I had to do on her chart. She went to the door behind me and opened it.

Suddenly she let out a huge wallop! "JERREEEEEEEEE!" she screamed at the top of her lungs.

I jumped out of my chair. She sounded like one of those mountain callers who sent messages over mountain ranges.

She turned and walked quietly to her chair and sat down again. "He'll be here shortly," she said to me.

Soon I heard trampling on the porch and Jerry walked in, pulling off his boots at the door. He was a large, robust man with flaming red cheeks from being out in the cold. He apologized for not coming in sooner but a cow was calving and he didn't want to leave her alone. I assured him that I understood. He settled down and I explained my service to them.

We went upstairs to their bedroom for the last part of my visit, the physical exam. It's no easy feat doing physical exams in people's homes. Doing pap smears and pelvic exams on a variety of beds from rollaways to waterbeds has made me appreciate my office. In Elvira's home, I put two chairs at the foot of her bed for her feet while I sat on a turned over wastebasket at the edge of her bed to do her pap smear.

It was late when I finished the exam. As I turned my back to put away all of my instruments, I heard her murmur that she wanted to put on her robe because she was going to bed soon. When I turned around, I couldn't believe my eyes. Elvira had made an amazing transformation. There she stood with a lavender see-through negligee with a revealingly low neckline. Her long hair tumbled loosely around her shoulders and down to her waist. I was speechless.

I must have stared at her for longer than I should. I looked away and quickly collected my thoughts. "Well, let's make an appointment for your next visit," I stammered.

I giggled to myself as I drove home in the cool night air. My job is never boring.

Because I covered a wide geographical area, I was always searching for more back-up physicians. Because of the restrictions on nurse-midwives, I was forced into begging doctors to work with me. I developed a schedule for myself so I could tolerate this degrading and emotionally exhausting exercise. After initiating one meeting with a doctor, I would give myself a three-week break before initiating another one. This would give me ample breaks between doctors and their rejections.

One day when I came home, I was surprised to hear the voice of Dr. Whitehall, a local obstetrician, on my answering machine. I hadn't yet contacted him because I knew that the group of doctors he was practicing with didn't like midwives.

I called his office, and his secretary put him on the line.

He was interested in meeting me, he told me. He was curious about my practice and wondered if we might be able to work out an arrangement where we could work together. I made an appointment to see him.

I hung up the phone, numb with disbelief. I had never been contacted by a doctor who wanted to work with me. This was amazing. I didn't quite understand this turn of events.

The day came to meet with Dr. Whitehall. It was cold and cloudy. I went to the office and told the secretary who I was.

"He's got three more patients to see," she said. "He'll be with you in ten minutes."

I sat down in the spacious waiting room. Immediately a nurse poked her head through the door and called two expectant mothers from the waiting room back to the examination rooms. Another mother was coming out of the examination rooms into the waiting room. About five minutes later one of the other mothers came back into the waiting room and went up to the receptionist to make an appointment.

"Boy, that was fast," the first mother said. She was still waiting to make a payment.

"Yeah, snap, in and out, just like that," the second mother answered. With a short laugh she added, "That's the way it should be!"

"Oh, I don't know," the first mother said. "I would have liked to have more time to ask some questions!"

I was shocked that the first woman was already finished with her appointment in such a short time.

I was called back to the office.

Dr. Whitehall was sitting behind his desk when I walked in. He rose to greet me, reached across the desk to shake my hand and invited me to sit down. He was a tall, lanky man. He was pleasant but cool. There was tension in his face and his thin lips seemed foreign to laughter.

The conversation was trivial at first. Then I decided to bite the bullet as soon as I could. I told him about my service. I explained about nurse-midwives, our training, certification, practice and legal relationship with physicians.

"So," I concluded, "one of the important things I need to practice is a physician who is willing to consult with my patients in the event that their pregnancies need medical attention."

"I'll be happy to do that," he said.

I couldn't believe my ears. How could this be? I had been used to thinking that obstetricians were against nurse-midwives and here was one of them offering to consult with my patients. I was amazed.

I gave him my protocols and arranged that my clients would come to meet him at the beginning of the pregnancy and then see him again once more toward the end of the pregnancy.

"Will your partners agree to your arrangement with me?" I ventured to ask.

He shrugged his shoulders. "I'll handle them," he answered.

"So, you'll be on call all the time for my clients?" I persisted.

"Yep," he murmured and held up his hand in dismissal.

I really didn't know what to think as I walked out of his office. I was suspicious. Maybe he was trying to prove something to his partners. Maybe he wanted a nurse-midwife to work for him, and this, to him, was a step in that direction. He seemed to accept it when I told him I wanted to work *with* a doctor, not *for* a doctor.

"Oh well," I thought to myself. "All I can do is send a few clients to him and see what happens."

I sent two families to him. Both of them reported that he was pleasant at their visit and assured them that he would be available if they needed him.

The months moved on. Then I got a client who had had a cesarean at another hospital and desperately wanted to try a vaginal birth. Kim felt strongly that she had been mismanaged at her previous birth. For this pregnancy, she was seeing Dr. Whitehall.

Midway through her pregnancy, Kim decided that to increase her chances of having a vaginal birth, she would have a midwife come with her to the hospital to give her support during labor and delivery. She asked Dr. Whitehall and the other physicians in the group if it would be okay and they all said it would be fine. That's when I came on the scene.

Kim came to see me a few times, and she and her husband came together for some childbirth education teaching. She gave me reports of her prenatal visits. For the most part, everything seemed to be going smoothly.

Then, toward the end of her pregnancy, Dr. Whitehall told her, "Don't expect that just because you have a midwife with you that you'll be protected from having a cesarean."

I should have been more concerned about this comment than I was, but I tried to reason with myself that he was merely giving her appropriate information. Sometimes women need a cesarean no matter who is with them. I played down Kim's rising concerns about how supportive the physicians were about her plans. I was wrong.

One beautiful morning Kim called me in labor. She had been laboring all night but now the contractions were getting closer. I told her to come to my house and I would check her before we went to the hospital. This had been discussed with her doctors and they had agreed to this plan. When she arrived, she was eight centimeters dilated and the baby was engaged in her pelvis. Her contractions were coming every two minutes and were quite strong. We called the hospital. Dr. Whitehall was on call and the birthing room was open but they were filling up with patients so we decided to go immediately. I still shudder at that decision.

During her prenatal care, Kim had told me that she was frightened of hospitals, but I had underestimated that fear. We arrived at the hospital and Dr. Whitehall checked her immediately. He announced that she was four centimeters dilated with the baby's head floating (not engaged in the pelvis). I was floored. I knew I couldn't have been that far off, but now that we were in the hospital, I couldn't do any hands-on care. I couldn't check behind him.

Kim was deflated. As the nurses went through their admitting routine, her contractions slowed considerably. They were now about ten minutes apart. Kim's brow was furrowed and when I asked her questions her answers were distracted. I tried to keep her on target, but the admitting area was busy and it was hard for me to interfere for the first half hour. When I finally got to Kim, I worked on getting her back on course. Dr. Whitehall came in again. His manner was curt and distant. He barely looked at me and barked out orders to the nurse. I got the distinct feeling I wasn't welcome. I tried to be friendly with him, and when he was at the nurse's desk I went out to try to strike up a conversation while the nurse finished admitting Kim.

"How do you think she'll do?" I asked him.

He looked at me for the first time. "I don't know," he said. "We'll give her a few more hours and see what she does."

"A few hours," I thought to myself. "What does that mean? At the rate her contractions were going now, she wouldn't be anywhere in a few hours."

I decided to change the subject. I could tell something was amiss. He was so abrupt and he would hardly look at me. Then it dawned on me: If she had a vaginal delivery, he would perceive it as my success. He didn't want it to look like midwives could be successful doing something that doctors had said was impossible.

"How do you like the two families I sent to you?" I asked.

"They're fine."

All too short an answer for my comfort.

The phone rang. He was called downstairs to the operating room. He turned on his heels, dismissing me with a hurried gesture and left the desk.

I was relieved he was gone. Now to get back to business. I went into the room and started an intense cheering section. I had to get her psyched up. She was like a wilted flower. I got her up. We walked. I put her in the shower. I made her stimulate her nipples to encourage contractions to come.

The nurse was sympathetic. She encouraged us and she came by to check on us between her other tasks. Over the two hours Dr. Whitehall was gone, we got her contractions back to every five minutes but she was pensive, fearful and jumpy. She kept saying, "He's going to come back soon."

Her fear was overwhelming. I felt sorry that I had underestimated it prenatally. I made a mental note to always discuss my clients' fears with them before they deliver.

Dr. Whitehall was gone longer than we expected. However he called an hour after he left and asked the nurse to check Kim vaginally. "Eight to nine centimeters," she announced. I knew then that I had been right. She had always been eight centimeters dilated because with the weak and irregular contractions she was having, her cervix couldn't possibly have gone from four to eight centimeters in one and a half hours. Kim was in the shower when Dr. Whitehall returned.

The nurse came into the bathroom. "He wants her out now," she said. "He wants to check her." She rolled her eyes at me, warning me that he was in a bad mood.

Kim had actually started to sound a little more positive before Dr. Whitehall returned. Her contractions were picking up slowly and she was feeling encouraged. We dried her off and went to the birthing room.

I sat in the back of the room watching him prepare to do the vaginal. I felt like time was standing still. Kim looked at me. I winked at her and gave her a thumbs up sign. She smiled.

The nurse put some lubricating gel on the doctor's gloved fingers. He leaned over my client and put his fingers in her vagina. I motioned to her to relax and breathe evenly. He worked his fingers up into her. I saw him getting progressively more forceful. Finally his whole hand was inside her. Kim started sweating. Suddenly she cried out in pain. I saw him jab upward forcefully. Her head jerked upward on her pillow. She grabbed onto the sides of the bed for support. Could he be pushing the baby up? I became alarmed. He wasn't stopping! This was like some of the vaginal exams I had watched Dr. Pima do in my old nursing days.

My fears were confirmed. He did not want Kim to have a vaginal delivery. After what seemed like an eternity, he took his fingers out of her vagina.

"She's not going anywhere," he announced, peeling his bloodied glove off his hand. "There's been absolutely no progress."

He barked orders to the nurse.

"Call anesthesiology," he ordered. "Let's get her ready for a section."

He turned to Kim. "You gave it your best shot," he said to her. "You can wait a little longer if you want, but there's been no progress and it doesn't look like there will be. If you go much longer, the baby could get in trouble. It's your decision, but I refuse to take responsibility for the outcome if you decide to wait."

He walked out of the room.

Kim was deflated. Her psyche was knocked down. Her contractions had all but stopped.

"I'm sorry, Juliana," she said to me. "I can't do it anymore."

I held her hand while they prepared her for surgery.

During the cesarean I sat out in the hall alone, waiting to hear whether she had a boy or girl. I was numb and couldn't quite sort out my thoughts. All I knew was that this was wrong.

After a while Dr. Whitehall walked out. "She had a boy," he called over to me as he scurried down the hall. "You all tried the best you could," he added over his shoulder. "But, she just couldn't do it." He disappeared around the corner.

The nurse who worked with us was pregnant. She wanted to have her baby at home. I started to see her for prenatal care. During one of our visits we talked about Dr. Whitehall.

I told her how horrified I was at his vaginal exam and that I thought that he pushed the baby back up into her pelvis.

"She didn't stand a chance with Dr. Whitehall," the nurse told me. Then she snickered, "We don't call him 'Roto Rooter' for nothing!"

A month later I received a call from Dr. Whitehall's office manager.

"May I please speak to Mrs. Fehr?" the woman's voice said.

"Speaking," I answered.

"This is Dr. Whitehall's office manager," she said. "He has asked me to inform you that he does not want to associate with your clients anymore."

I wasn't surprised at this development. What surprised me was that he didn't call himself but had his office manager do it. I thought he had more decency than that, or at least more courage. I have no respect for anyone who can't do their own dirty work.

"That's interesting," I responded thoughtfully to her statement. "I wonder why he's not calling me and got you to do it instead."

She stumbled over her response to this unexpected observation.

"Oh," she said haltingly, "He's, uh, very busy, and, uh, he just wanted you to know right when he made his decision."

"Well, I would appreciate it if you would give him the message that I would like to talk to him. Please have him give me a call at his earliest convenience."

"I'll give him the message," she said.

Of course he never called, but I had another way to get him to take responsibility for his actions. I called my two clients whom he had agreed to be back up for and told them of his decision. Because it was very close to their due dates, they were outraged.

One of them, Linda, called him up and demanded to speak with him. He told her that he didn't remember her and he never told her that he would be her back-up physician. She told him that she would notify her lawyer of this interaction.

My second client called him a few hours later and he immediately told her that he was still backing her up. He called Linda back that afternoon and told her he would be her back-up physician.

I called Dr. Peterson and told him of the turn of events. He chuckled and assured me that he would be the backup.

I will never know why Dr. Whitehall got himself into this situation. I suspected that he was playing some little internal political game with his partners and when the going got a little rough, he turned in his cards. His political game could have threatened the health of my patients and their babies. And, because I was subservient to him, my hands were tied while I watched him do it.

But I wasn't to be tied for long. I was already tired of my "marriage" to doctors and I wanted a divorce. The relationship between doctors and midwives could indeed be hostile and as it stood now midwives were the victims in the fight. The legislature was not on our side, so our chapter of the ACNM was spurred into action to fight for our survival.

In early January I became chairperson of the chapter, a post that I would keep for the next four years. My major goal was to increase our professional profile in the state. We needed to keep abreast of developments all over the state regarding nurse-midwifery practice. To do that effectively, we needed more nurse-midwives to join the chapter. As it was, our membership was hopelessly small and the attendance at chapter meetings was abysmal. There were too few active nurse-midwives and we were spread out over a large state. Most of us couldn't travel a long distance because we had families dependent on us or we had to be on call for patients.

At the first meeting I chaired, four of us (the only four who could show up) had a meeting around the kitchen table at a midwife's home. We had gotten hold of a letter put out by the Virginia Obstetrical and Gynecological Society that had a note at the bottom reminding members to come up with agenda items for their next meeting in the Bahamas. Having their business meeting in the Bahamas was the main ingredient to a group's survival. No one was going to turn down the chance to take a trip to the Bahamas as a tax deductible business expense. No wonder they had a good turnout for their meetings. Well, I was not going to let our business meetings fall apart. I was not to be thwarted by the many obstacles in my path. Very early in my term as chairperson, I developed the "conference call chapter meeting." To make it easier for midwives to attend, we started having our quarterly chapter meeting by conference call. What I was lacking in money, I made up for in determination and I was determined to start our divorce proceedings. Not only did we have conference calls, but I attended every meeting in the state that had anything to do with maternal-infant health and nurse-midwives.

Meanwhile, the babies kept coming and my service seemed to take me to some of the far corners of the rural areas I served. Not only was the radius of my service area large (one hour's drive from my home in all directions), but the people I serviced were unique. At the beginning of the year I had a home visit to do. Jean was a wonderful woman who lived out in the country and was expecting her first baby. When she gave me directions to her home, I knew I was going to be in an isolated area. Her directions went something like this: Turn right onto the road at the grocery store, go about two miles and turn right on the dirt road after the bridge. Turn right at the fork and keep going even though the road looks like it isn't. Go till you can't go anymore and you'll see a road going up the mountain to the left. Keep going up until you see a gate on your left (don't make any right turns because you'll just go down a steep incline and you won't be able to get back up). Make a left past the gate and go until you see a broken down old truck. Past that is an old oak tree. (I tried to remember what an oak tree looked like!) Turn onto that road and that will eventually end in our yard. There are three big dogs who will bark at you, but don't mind them because they're friendly.

As it turned out, I arrived at her house in one piece amidst a chorus of barking dogs. She came out to greet me and led me into her home. Jean and her husband Shaun had built their own home and it was quite cozy. Jean was a naturalist to the maximum extent. They had no running water and no electricity, and there was no indoor plumbing. When I say these words, most people conjure up an image of a ramshackle home with poor people living inside. Not true. Jean and Shaun made a deliberate choice to live in this manner. Their lights operated on propane fuel and they had a propane refrigerator. Their house was solar heated, supplemented with wood. Their bath was outside and heated with wood underneath. Their water came from a spring.

The living room was comfortable and sunny. Two walls were lined with books. Their bedroom was in a loft. They were by no means poor, but they were committed to living out their ideals. The kitchen was rustic but immaculate, with a variety of herbs hanging from the ceiling to dry. Fresh baked bread was on the counter and homemade jams were nearby. She had a wood stove for cooking as well as heating.

After the visit I left with ambivalent feelings. It might be a perfect birth—just what everyone imagines a home birth to be—but if the weather was inclement, it could be terrible if I had an emergency and couldn't get through their road.

"Well, Juliana," I thought to myself. "You chose to be a rural midwife and this is what you get."

Just as I feared, it started snowing heavily during Jean's labor. She delivered a little boy in the early morning hours up in the warm cozy loft by candlelight. Shaun was supporting her in his arms when the baby was born. It was a perfect birth.

I stayed with them overnight and by the time daylight came, the snow was ten inches deep. I worried about going down the steep mountain road, but I wanted to go home before it got worse. Waving goodbye, I resolutely steered my four-wheel-drive car down the hill. Surprisingly, the road was better with the freshly fallen snow on it. There were no more terrible potholes. I drove home resolving to write a commercial about how dependable my car was.

The next baby I delivered was born to a couple who were deeply religious. Betty believed that the Lord would carry her through the labor and birth.

Betty was quiet during her labor. When her contractions came she would look at me and then close her eyes to breathe through them. I enjoyed watching her and stayed nearby to monitor the baby and give her an added sense of security. Time was measured by her contractions. They were like a ticking clock. I have often mused that I could set my clock by the regularity of some women's contractions.

Finally after a particularly long contraction, Betty lifted her head, looked at me and said, "I think I might be ready to push now."

I smiled at her. "Go ahead and push very gently with the next contraction if you feel the urge."

Her next contraction came. She groaned. A deep, soft, low groan. She was gently bearing down with her groan.

She sat quietly to wait for the next one.

Another deep groan. It was a little longer this time.

The room came alive. Relatives scurried around getting cameras ready and holding other children. My birth assistant brought my equipment closer and handed me my gloves and instruments.

Betty moved to the edge of the bed. The baby's head was showing.

"The baby has lots of hair," I exclaimed.

Everyone rushed over to take a look

"It's so dark," her sister said.

Betty didn't say anything. She was concentrated inward. I knew she wouldn't say anything else until the baby was born. Her husband stroked her hair and wiped her forehead with a wet cloth.

The baby's head was born slowly. The rest of its body slid out easily.

"It's a boy," her husband said.

Betty was laughing and crying at the same time. There wasn't a dry eye in the room. She held the baby in her arms.

I watched her with admiration. How strong and focused she was. I could only be grateful that I was able to be with her at this moment.

On my way home I was overwhelmed by fatigue. These two births were right together and I needed a rest.

"But, wait a minute," I said aloud to myself. "Now that Betty delivered two weeks early, I'm free for three weeks before I have to be on call for my April births. I'm going to go to Holland to see my parents."

My mind started buzzing. In a flash I calculated my trip.

"I could leave the day after tomorrow and be there for over two weeks. I'll call my parents tomorrow morning, do my postpartum visits, get my tickets and be on the plane the next morning," I thought.

My plan completely dispelled my fatigue. I was so happy to think that I would see my mother again. I knew that she would be overjoyed. I rushed home and started my preparations.

The next day was filled with bustling activity. I had called my parents and they were thrilled. I hurried to my clients' homes and did their postpartum visits. I arranged to have another midwife answer questions my clients might have while I was gone. Their consulting physicians would see them in an emergency. The last thing I had to do was go to the bank and get money to pay for the tickets. That's when the bomb dropped.

As I walked in the door of the bank, my beeper went off. I called home. Eric answered.

"What's the matter?" I asked.

"Juliana," he said slowly. I knew something was terribly wrong.

"David just called. Your sister Willemien has been in a serious car accident."

The breath was knocked out of me. I sank down into the chair behind the desk of one of the bank workers.

"Is she alive?" I barely breathed into the phone. I started trembling all over.

"Yes," he said, "but David says there were some head injuries so they don't know yet how she'll pull out of it."

"What happened?" I asked. I felt so panicked I didn't know what to do.

I felt like dropping the phone and running away. Down the street. Miles away. I didn't know where. I didn't care.

"I don't know, Honey," Eric said. "I've got his number. Give him a call and he can tell you everything."

I hung up and slowly dialed my sister's number.

Dave answered. "Willie is being transferred to the University hospital in Burlington," he told me. "She's had some pretty serious internal bleeding. She's conscious now and then. They have her on a respirator. It's pretty touch-and-go. I can't talk anymore because I have to go. I'll call reports to my mother and you can call her later." He hung up.

I put down the phone and stared numbly out of the window.

"At least she's alive. At least she's alive." I kept repeating to myself.

My trembling slowed. I needed to figure out what to do. Should I go to my sister or should I go to my mother? If I went to my sister, I would be there if she needed me or to hold vigil by her bedside. I've always believed that having loved ones close by aids the healing process. On the other hand, I knew her convalescence and recovery would be long. Wouldn't it be better to be with my mother to soften the blow and help her through the next two weeks?

I called David back. He was already gone. His mother answered the phone.

"Go to your mother," she said. "She will need you these two weeks."

So it was settled. I spent the next two weeks in Holland. My parents and I held our vigil by the phone. Luckily, good fortune was on our side. After the first harrowing days the reports began looking more positive. Each day progress was made and after two weeks we were all relieved that her injuries were no longer life threatening and her head injuries didn't cause any damage.

I was glad to have been able to be there with my mother through this time but as the end of my visit approached, I started dreading leaving her and wondered why I put myself through this anguish. I often felt like I had to have a few days to recuperate after leaving my mother so far behind.

As I said goodbye to them at the airport, I wondered what they would do if I just grabbed them, fell to the ground and insisted on staying with them. I remember doing that in the first grade when my mother brought me to my classroom and I took an instant dislike to my teacher. I walked into the room, fell on the floor and screamed until my mother agreed to sit in the back of the room. When she got up to leave after I seemed to be settled in my desk, I would scream again. Now, even though I was a grown woman, I wasn't immune to that familiar flash of desperation that stabbed my heart. But, I kissed them and turned away to board the plane. Again, I left Holland in a veil of tears as the plane taxied down the runway. My children held my hands.

I knew that my intense emotions upon leaving my mother were remnants of the old "separation anxiety" I had as a child. One of my mother's favorite stories was how she wasn't allowed to hold me until twelve hours after I was born. When I was finally in her arms, she discovered a little pink bow taped to my bald head. He first words to me were, "Let me look at you," and immediately I waved my arms in response to her voice. She would smile when telling me the story, but when I asked her why I was away from her for so long, she would merely furrow her eyebrows and shrug her shoulders. In her previous home deliveries in Holland she had never been separated from her babies. Things were just different in America.

My mother's story about our first separation must have influenced me deeply because I know that my unwillingness to separate from my loved ones has influenced my behavior as a mother and my philosophies as a midwife. And, just as I wouldn't compromise with anyone about leaving my mother when I was in first grade or leaving my children in day care now, I won't compromise about separating mothers and babies at birth. Hospital personnel don't have to take a baby away from its mother to "monitor" him. They can do that right in the mother's room. But I find it ironic that, even when hospitals have allowed mothers and babies to stay together, now mothers are insisting that their babies be taken to the nursery. I'm sad to see that somehow mothers have been convinced to start practicing separation behaviors right at the beginning.

But why do I think it's so vital that mothers and babies aren't separated at all after birth? Because bonding ensures the survival of the child, the mother and their long-term relationship. In fact, the bonding behavior is a fail-safe set of acts occurring in both mother and infant that serve to lock the mother and infant together. An alert and undrugged mother who delivers in the upright position in a supportive environment is a wonder to watch. She and her infant start to secure their relationship immediately. When she first touches her baby, she turns her head to align her eyes with his. As their eyes meet, she raises the pitch of her voice to soothe his cries. His ears are tuned to high pitched sounds and he stops in response to her voice and starts to search for her face. When his crying slows, his blood pressure and intracranial pressure go down to normal levels.

After the mother's first tenuous touches she brings her baby to her breast, usually the left breast, the one over her heart. His cheek then brushes her nipple and he turns his head and opens his mouth to start to suck. His nuzzling against her nipple causes her to release oxytocin, a powerful hormone that contracts her uterus to stop her from bleeding too much. The oxytocin also contracts her milk ducts to push the pre-milk, colostrum, out to her nipples. Simultaneously, her body also releases prolactin, another hormone that causes her breasts to start producing milk.

As they are together and the mother is looking down at her baby, the smell of his body (very pleasant) causes her to release antibodies into her breastmilk to protect him from bacteria in his environment. Finally, the heat she releases from her body keeps him warm and active.

Studies point to a sensitive period for human parents during the first hours of life. Indeed, for the first 60 to 90 minutes, the infant, if alert, is responsive and especially appealing. As Marshall Klaus, a renowned pediatrician, says, "The infant's broad array of sensory and motor abilities evoke responses from the mother and begin the communication which may be especially helpful for attachment." Parents and infants who are deprived of this time may have difficulty attaching to each other. This doesn't mean that mothers and infants who are separated can't make up for it, but if there is such a sensitive period, why not let them take advantage of it? In a society where abuse, neglect and separation run rampant, it certainly can't hurt.

As always, my work eased the pain of leaving my mother. My office hours were getting hectic and I often found myself busy from morning to evening on all three days. I still did my first prenatal visits at home and, because I always schedule an hour for my appointments, a home visit was quite a time commitment.

One of my home visits that spring was quite interesting. When Lavinia called me she told me that she was having her eleventh baby. As she put it, her ninth baby was born in the hospital elevator and her tenth was born in the lobby, so why go in at all? I explained to her the increased risk of having so many babies and told her that I couldn't do her delivery unless I had adequate medical backup. As it was, I told her that I wouldn't commit to anything until after I had done a complete history and physical.

We made our appointment. I was surprised at what I saw when I drove up to her home. There in front of me was a beautiful mansion. It was so large that when I went home, I teased Eric that if I moved in I'd still be a half an hour away from her. I knocked on the front door. Lavinia answered and showed me to the third living room to the right. Actually, I think it was the family room because it had a bar and a TV.

I sat with her on the couch and asked her all of the questions I needed. She was a nervous woman who acted slightly impatient with all of my questions. Of course, it got long and drawn out when we got to the history of her pregnancies. Her two youngest children were running in and out of the room and finally they trotted away with the housekeeper. I did her physical exam on the couch. We postponed the pap smear for the next visit at my office.

She was in excellent physical shape. She was aware of the right foods and she swam a mile a day in their pool. She had help with her children and someone else cleaned the house. In fact, several of her children were away at preparatory school. Her obstetrician was a good family friend and he said that he would be her backup for the birth. I also arranged to have Dr. Petersen be her backup.

Her prenatal course was marked by appointment cancellations. After three of them, I insisted on talking to both her and her husband. On the morning I arrived to meet Robert, I realized that he knew nothing about midwives and she hadn't attempted to tell him. All he knew was that Lavinia wanted to have her baby at home and she had hired a midwife to help her. He grudgingly agreed to meet me only because I told her I wouldn't deliver her baby if he didn't.

Robert was in "his" chair. He didn't bother to rise when I entered the room, and he waved me to a place on the couch next to Lavinia. I recognized immediately what was going on. This man was treating me as if he was interviewing an applicant for a position on his domestic staff. I decided to sit back and enjoy the conversation. I had only read about this kind of interview in Gothic romances. This was going to be fun.

"So, Lavinia wants to have her baby at home," Robert began. "And, I suppose you can help her do that. I really don't agree with her about this but I suppose it's her body so it's up to her."

He eyed me carefully behind his nonchalant facade. I could tell immediately that he loved her very much. He was truly concerned about her but he didn't want to show it.

I decided that I needed to be straightforward with him.

"I want you to know that I can't guarantee that I will deliver your baby at home. I have stringent guidelines for determining who is appropriate for a home birth. Lavinia must keep in the low-risk category throughout her pregnancy for me to deliver her baby," I explained.

Robert looked surprised. He leaned back and surveyed me behind the smoke of his cigarette.

"You seem like an intelligent woman," he commented. "What made you become a midwife?"

I saw that he was befuddled by the situation he was in. He was expecting a midwife circa Prissy in *Gone with the Wind,* and he was faced with me talking about "protocols," "low-risk" and "high-risk."

I started to explain to him how I had changed my career from teaching to midwifery.

"So," I said after telling him about my teaching experience, "I went back to school to get a bachelor's degree in nursing so I could become a midwife."

"You mean," he interrupted, "you have a bachelor's degree from college?"

"Oh yes," I assured him. "In fact I have two bachelor's degrees, one in special education and one in nursing. I also have a master's degree in midwifery."

Robert's eyes widened. "A master's degree!" he exclaimed. "What school did you go to?"

"I got my bachelor's degree in nursing from the University of Virginia and my master's degree in midwifery from Georgetown University."

He leaned forward in his chair. All of his nonchalance disappeared. This man was obviously surprised.

"Georgetown! That's my alma mater!"

"Oh really," I said. "What did you do there?"

"I got my bachelor's degree in business," he said. He jumped up from his chair and went to the bar. "Would you like a drink?" he asked. "Really, we have anything you want; coke, juice, wine. You probably don't drink alcohol at this time of day anyway."

I smiled to myself.

"What year did you graduate from Georgetown?" he called as he was preparing his drink.

We had an easy conversation about school and a variety of other subjects. Robert was very curious about midwifery, especially the politics. I told him everything he wanted to know.

As I got up to leave, he offered me some advice.

"Lavinia is stubborn and doesn't like to follow anyone's advice," he said as he looked at her in a loving, reproachful way.

Lavinia maintained her silence.

"She's going to be awful to give prenatal care to."

She denied his charges. "I'll do everything Juliana says," she exclaimed.

She hesitated for a moment. "I do so hate traveling such a long distance to your office though. Would you mind coming here for prenatal visits if we paid you for your time?"

So it was settled. I did the rest of the prenatal visits at her home, in the family room.

When the day of her delivery arrived, Robert called me at 2:00 A.M. "Lavinia is in labor now and she's going to have her baby soon," he reported.

I rushed to their home. On the way it dawned on me that I didn't know where her bedroom was. In an average house that's not a problem, but in a house the size of theirs, it definitely could present a challenge. I had to laugh at myself. All of those prenatal visits and I didn't think to ask where their bedroom was.

I arrived at the house and pulled up to the front door I always used. I tried the lock. It was open. I pushed the door open and quickly put my equipment in the foyer. I cupped my hands around my mouth.

"I'm here," I called. My voice seemed to echo through the large, still house.

"We're up here," I heard a voice call from upstairs.

"Tell me where to come," I called out.

I followed the directions up the stairs and entered their master bedroom. Lavinia was lying on her side on the bed. Robert was holding her leg up.

"I think the baby is coming," he said.

I rushed to their side of the massive bed. Indeed, the baby's head was beginning to present. I guided Robert's hands to cup the baby's head and encouraged her to stop pushing as I pulled on my gloves.

Their baby's head slid out right into Robert's hands. I felt a cord around the neck. I tried to pull it around the baby's head, but it was too tight. I quickly clamped the cord in two places and cut in between. The rest of the baby slid out into Robert's hands. He started crying immediately. Robert was holding him, dumfounded that he had delivered him. After spending the rest of the morning celebrating the baby's birth with a father who couldn't wipe the ear-to-ear grin off his face, I left with a new lesson learned: Don't ever assume you know where bedrooms are.

During the spring of 1985, I dedicated some time to building up my gynecology caseload. I put some advertisements in the paper and I contacted some members of Rosemont, West Virginia. I offered to come to someone's house and, if a group of women came, I would do all of their pap smears. The first of these events was successful. I went to a woman's home and about ten women arrived. They brought over some snacks and took some time to socialize while I did pap smears and breast exams. A lot of women commented on how comfortable they felt with this kind of arrangement. My message to them was: "You are not sick. You are just taking preventive health steps." Many women who came hadn't had pap smears for many years because they felt intimidated going to the doctor's office for this exam.

It was in the spring that I first had to transfer a client to the hospital. Debbie was a twenty-year-old woman having her first baby. Her boyfriend,

Jack, was in his late thirties. He had two children from his previous marriage who were living with them. Debbie struggled throughout her pregnancy to be a mother to two children who were almost half her age. It was hard on her. Jack also was very demanding. He was very set in his ways, and if he defined something as "wrong," he was formidable. One good point was that he was very conscious of nutrition and had a healthy lifestyle. His inflexibility, however, made life hard for her, and I know that she enjoyed sneaking a taco at the local Mexican restaurant after her visits with me.

Early one morning Debbie called me with contractions that were twenty to thirty minutes apart. We kept in touch throughout most of the day and by night they were every ten minutes. My birth assistant and I arrived at her home late at night. She and Jack were on their bed. He was very loving toward her as she breathed rhythmically through her contractions. My birth assistant and I watched them.

Debbie's face was childlike, almost angelic. She was trying so hard. Jack was behind her, holding her in his arms. I could tell that he was more experienced, having watched his ex-wife give birth to their two children.

At first, Debbie's baby's heart rate was stable through her contractions. If the baby's heart rate gets slower during the contractions, it might be a sign of fetal distress.

I listened to the baby's heartbeat frequently. Usually for a labor going at Debbie's pace, I listen every fifteen minutes. As a labor gets more intense, however, I listen more frequently. It was when Debbie's contractions got to five minutes apart that I started hearing a problem. I was listening every ten minutes when I helped her to the toilet. When we got back I listened and detected a drop in the heart rate during the contraction. By the end of the contraction the rate went back up again. The drop was slight so I put her on her left side and listened again. (Sometimes changing a mother's position can eliminate a deceleration in her baby's heartbeat.) The drop was more pronounced.

"The baby's heartbeat has a slight deceleration during your contractions," I told her quietly.

After being through my Emergencies and Complications lecture, they knew what I meant.

"I'm going to keep changing your position to see if I can rectify it."

A few more contractions went by. I put her in a "hands and knees" position, a standing position and on her right side. No position helped.

I knew from the nature of the deceleration that it was probably a problem with the baby's umbilical cord. It was either around the baby's neck or somehow tangled around the baby. Usually this kind of deceleration isn't a problem as long as it doesn't worsen or get too low. But definitely, in a series of about four to five contractions, Debbie's baby's heartrate was going too low.

As gently and as rapidly as I could, I prepared Debbie for transport to the hospital.

"I really think that the baby's heartbeat is going too low for me to feel comfortable keeping you at home to deliver. I'm not real sure what's causing the heartbeat to go down but I think the umbilical cord might be compressed."

I kept my voice low and calm. I didn't want to alarm them but at the same time I wanted to emphasize the necessity of transfer. It had crossed my mind that Jack, being so committed to alternatives and so scornful of the medical system, might balk at transferring to the hospital.

I was wrong. He was very cooperative and he joined us in getting Debbie to the hospital as quickly as possible.

I administered oxygen to Debbie during the drive to the hospital. We transferred her to Dr. Moore. When we arrived at the hospital, we went directly to labor and delivery. The nurse put the fetal monitor around Debbie's abdomen. Sure enough, the heartbeat was decelerating during the contractions. Even though it went down pretty low, it came up nicely right after the contraction.

I stayed at Debbie's side. "Breathe evenly and slowly," I told her. "Stay focused on your labor. Breathe deeply and give the baby plenty of oxygen."

My whispers must have sounded urgent because she looked at me intensely and said, "Don't leave me. Stay right here next to me."

"I'm right here," I assured her.

Dr. Moore came into the room. He looked at the monitor strip and did a vaginal exam. She was nine centimeters dilated.

"Let's keep her laboring for awhile," he said to me. "It looks like we might have a cord around the neck, but since the heartbeat is coming up nicely, I think we can let her try to push this baby out."

I worked with her for another hour before she got the urge to push. We were there together, Jack, Debbie, me and my birth assistant. We were quiet. The only sound in the room was the beeping of the baby's heartbeat on the fetal monitor. It was eerie listening to it slow down during the contractions. It seemed to teeter momentarily at the peak of the contraction and then it would speed up again. We all exchanged pensive glances as we listened to it and watched Debbie struggle to maintain control at the peak of her contractions. I adjusted her oxygen mask. Dr. Moore came in frequently to check the monitor strip.

With her first push I knew that we could go on no longer. We needed to get the baby out fast. I went out to the hallway to get Dr. Moore. He was sitting at the nurse's desk.

"She's starting to bear down involuntarily now," I told him. "The baby's heartbeat is really slowing at the peak of her contractions and I feel that it would be a good idea to get the baby out soon."

"Let's see what's going on," he said as he heaved himself out of the chair. I had forgotten what a big man he was.

The heartbeat was at a low point when we walked back in the room. He studied the monitor strip awhile and put on his glove to do a vaginal exam.

"She's complete," he said. That meant her cervix was completely dilated and she could push her baby out.

"Let's take her back to the delivery room and get this baby born."

I stepped around to stand next to Debbie. I leaned over and whispered to her. "Debbie, the baby's heartbeat is getting pretty slow during your contractions now. It's still going up nicely right after the peak of the contraction so we think the baby's okay. You're completely dilated and ready to push the baby out. It's real important that it gets born soon. I'll stay right with you and talk you through each contraction. I'll try to let you know everything Dr. Moore does as soon as he does it."

She nodded at me and squeezed my hand. Her eyes remained closed and her face was buried by the oxygen mask.

In the delivery room everything was set up to perform a vacuum extraction. We got Debbie up on the delivery table and tied her legs in the stirrups. Her contractions were coming very close together now.

"Push, Debbie," I spoke urgently to her. "Concentrate on pushing your baby out."

Jack held her up in a semireclining position while we waited for Dr. Moore to get ready. Everyone was scurrying around quietly. Dr. Moore came in. I focused on Debbie. When I heard him pull his stool up to the table I knew he was ready.

"Dr. Moore is going to cut an episiotomy now so he can help you deliver the baby," I told her. "You're going to feel a stinging sensation as he gives you the numbing medication for the episiotomy."

She jumped with the first shot.

"Breathe in and out," I told her. "Stay focused on the baby."

He pulled out his scissors and cut the episiotomy. The familiar sound of the snipping scissors seemed to echo in my brain.

Debbie seemed oblivious. She was pushing continually.

Dr. Moore put the vacuum extractor into Debbie's vagina and applied it to the baby's scalp.

I leaned down next to Debbie's face again.

"Dr. Moore is going to pull on the baby while you push," I said. "Be sure to push down in the direction that he's pulling. Work with him."

Dr. Moore started pulling.

"Push hard, Debbie, push hard." Jack was encouraging her in one ear and I in the other.

She pushed with all of her might. After what seemed like an eternity but was only a few moments, the baby was born. His cord was tangled all around him and he was bloody from her episiotomy. His little pale body hung limply as Dr. Moore suctioned him out. The cord was cut and the nurse took him over to the warmer.

His cries were muted little mews. The nurse continued to suction him. Jack and Debbie were holding each other and crying. I went over to watch the baby.

As the nurse and I stimulated him, his mews turned into howls.

"Is he all right? Is he all right?" Debbie asked.

"He's doing great," I answered.

Jack came over to look at him.

"Boy, he looks like he's been through a lot," he commented. Surely he was right. The baby's face was bruised and swollen from his journey.

We wrapped him up tight and brought him over to Debbie.

She cooed to him and tried to comfort him. The nurse came over and took him to the nursery.

I found myself cringing. More than ever this mother and baby needed to stay together. They had both had a traumatic time and they needed each other. The only reason the baby was going to the nursery was to go under the warmer to be monitored while he waited for the pediatrician to arrive. Why can't they warm the babies in the delivery room?

But these concerns were trivial now. Debbie and her baby had needed the medical system to come through this alive and well. They would have to live by the rules. Someday there would be hospitals where the providers would only perform emergency procedures and then teach the mother to provide the primary care. The mother and baby would be supported as a unit and taught to be independent and confident as they began their relationship.

I left the hospital that day grateful that Debbie and her baby were fine and that Dr. Moore had been so willing to help them. But I also left with the feeling that the system must be changed.

A few days after Debbie's delivery, another client, Nan, called me in labor.

I enjoyed Nan. She was a registered nurse and her husband, Hugh, was a photographer. They lived in the country and were building a little farm. Nan loved animals and had quite a variety of them. She owned horses, geese, a pitbull and a tarantula. In contrast to Debbie's birth, Nan's was fun. In fact, I don't think I've ever laughed as much at a birth as I did at this one.

It was a cold night, so Hugh had to bring the goslings in the kitchen to keep warm. Nan was upstairs getting some rest and Hugh went up to be with her. My birth assistant and I stayed downstairs and drank a cup of tea. As we idly gossiped, I saw something flash by out of the corner of my eye. Then another flash. Then another. I bent under the table and found the goslings all around my feet. Of course, as soon as they saw me, they ran away as fast as their little feet could carry them. They stumbled over each other and narrowly avoided trampling each other down as each fell on his face.

I smiled at them and watched them settle down as they got far enough away from me. Suddenly I noticed that there was a leader in this gosling crew and all of the goslings were copying their older sibling's movements exactly. When he drank water, they did. When he peeped, they did. When he spread his wings, so did they. It was such a comical sight that soon we were in tears laughing at them. They even bobbed their heads and stumbled when he did. Now I know where the term "silly goose" came from.

Eventually, they all settled down to sleep in a corner that their leader chose, and I went up to check on Nan. Her contractions had picked up and she was looking a little worried. In fact, she was almost agitated. I rubbed her back and spoke gently to her. Hugh was looking a little lost and helpless. I was having a hard time calming her down. She just didn't respond to me as easily as I thought she would. Suddenly Hugh came over and said, "Let me try." I was totally unprepared for the events that followed.

Hugh took control. He grabbed Nan's legs and started rubbing them vigorously. In fact, he operated almost like a vibrator. He started talking to her as if she were running a race and he was the announcer.

"Okay, Nan," he announced. "Another contraction is here and we're going to start. [Pause] OKAY, NOW! BREATHE! IN AND OUT AND IN AND OUT AND IN AND OUT AND IN AND OUT. YOU'VE GOT IT NOW BABY," he cheered. "IT'S MOVING ON NOW, IT'S MOVING! GO! GO! GO! GO!"

All the while he was rubbing and shaking her legs ferociously. My birth assistant looked at me with concern. "What's this guy doing?" her lips mouthed silently.

I shrugged my shoulders. I could hardly suppress a giggle.

Hugh went on, "Okay Nan, okay folks. The contraction's almost over. SHE'S FINISHED! ALL RIGHT! THAT'S GREAT! YOU DID IT!"

He reached over to wipe his face and take a sip of juice. He perched himself at her legs to get ready for the next contraction. Nan looked at him gratefully and smiled. They developed quite a system. She squeezed his hand when she felt the contraction starting and he started vibrating her legs and talking her through the race.

I chuckled to myself. Well, this certainly is a new method of psychoprophylaxis in childbirth. Nan was totally relaxed with him and he certainly was forceful about his technique.

I couldn't help laughing throughout the night. It was like "Sunday at the Races!" I spent my time monitoring the baby and bringing Hugh juice, a change of shirt when his got wet with sweat and a washcloth to wipe his face.

Early in the morning Nan delivered a beautiful little baby boy. The race was finally won. Hugh looked exultant in his sweat-soaked shirt. It was a sweet victory for them. Moments later he dropped exhausted to the bed and fell into a deep sleep.

Hours later, I left them all sleeping cozily in their bed. Hugh had not stirred through all of my exams and ministrations. I tucked Nan and her baby in, and gingerly walked past their pitbull and tarantula, pretending not to be afraid. The goslings scurried away as I walked past them in the kitchen and I drove down their bumpy road, out onto the highway and home to my wonderful bed.

It was time for me to penetrate the community again. This time I accepted an invitation to the local businesswomen's association to attend one of their meetings. I dressed in my finest and arrived at the meeting. The woman who invited me greeted me and showed me to my seat. She didn't sit with me but left me with a group of women at the table. We went through cursory introductions and then turned our attention to the meeting. I sat through discussions about minutes, agendas and future speakers. I listened to a fun talk given by their guest speaker about smocking.

After the formal meeting was over everyone socialized around coffee and donuts. A few women gathered around me and started asking questions. During these "question-and-answer periods" I always struggle to focus the conversation on midwifery and what we have to offer, but usually people start telling me birth stories that are so laden with fear, disappointment and hysteria that I find it hard to avoid pointing out the dangers of medical management. Particularly frustrating are statements such as these: "I (or my baby) would have died if we hadn't been in the hospital!" I want to tell them that many times medical management in hospitals create their own disasters. And, when I detect the guilt and anger hidden in their voices, I want to tell them they are not to blame. In fact, I want to tell them that no single person is at fault. Rather, the entire system must be changed. However, after talking to many women I have concluded that mothers must learn to resolve the negative feelings and guilt they have surrounding the births of their children even after "everything turns out fine," because it is the anger and guilt that forces women to "continue laboring" for many years after the births of their babies.

The conversation that night took the same course. I was extra careful with my answers because I knew that my audience was very conservative and not exactly willing to bust the system. At least I thought I knew that.

"Now, my daughter-in-law had her baby in a birthing room," said a grand-motherly woman. "She delivered naturally and said she really enjoyed it." Her voice droned on as she told me all about the experience. My mind started wandering. It was the end of a long day and I was tired. Unfortunately, I was giving her only half of my attention.

"I read in your ad in the newspaper that you do pap smears," she said.

"Yes," I answered.

"Well, let me tell you what happened with my last pap smear," she started.

"Oh no," I thought to myself. "I hope this story doesn't take too long."

She went on. "I was feeling inside my vagina and I felt a little bump, about the size of a BB, on my cervix."

That definitely caught my attention. I didn't expect to have a conversation like this here. I looked at the other women at the table. They were wide-eyed and quiet. Some murmured with embarrassment.

"I went to my doctor and told him to check it out," she continued, oblivious to her companions' discomfort. "He did a pap smear and told me it was nothing and sent me home. Well, I wasn't satisfied with his answer. Of course it was something, otherwise it wouldn't be there," she added em-phatically, pounding her fist on the table.

I suppressed an urge to giggle at the circumstance I was in. I was sitting at a table with a group of very conservative older women who apparently never talked of such intimate things, while one of them, obviously a bird of a different feather, was telling me all about her gynecological history in ex-cruciating detail.

Her story continued. "So, I went home and dug out a plastic speculum that I had picked up at a women's health fair a while back and I decided to take a look for myself."

A chair screeched against the floor as one of the table's occupants left. The others sat there numbly.

She went on, oblivious to her surroundings. "I put the speculum inside of me and got a flashlight and a mirror and took a look. Sure enough there it was. A little bump. I decided to watch it every month. After about three months it got bigger, so I went back to my doctor. He finally removed it but wouldn't talk to me very much about what it was. He just said it was nothing serious and waved me out of his office."

She looked around to all of our companions. "Can you imagine that this guy wouldn't even talk to me?" she exclaimed.

They all sat still, not responding.

"Now," she said, turning back to me. "Would you handle something like that?"

I kept as straight a face as I possibly could.

"I would do your pap smear and pelvic exam, and if I found anything that was out of the range of normal, I would refer you to my consulting physician," I explained. "I would always discuss my findings with you and explain his reports."

"Oh good," she said, leaning back in her chair. "I don't know about you girls," she said to her companions. "But, I'm going to start going to Juliana."

Our companions seemed to sigh with relief that our conversation had come to an end.

In the beginning of the summer I experienced one of the most trying deliveries of my career. The couple, Roberta and Ron, had contacted me at the beginning of the year. Early one January morning, while I was still in bed, Roberta first called. It was one of the most interesting calls I have received.

"Juliana? You don't know me, but I got your name from the paper," the voice on the other end of the line said. There was an urgency in her tone and her words came quickly as if she wanted to make sure she told me everything before I could say a word.

"I really don't know when I'm due because my cycles were thrown off when my husband and I got married," she said.

I got suspicious. Because it was before 7:00 A.M., I wondered if she was in labor and wanted me to attend her birth. I had already had people try to get me to come to their labors even though I didn't even know them.

"You see," she continued hurriedly, "my husband and I got married seven times in one month, and I know the excitement affected my ovulation. We were blessed with fertility by a lot of people who married us, so I think I ovulated a few times in one month."

I was just waiting for her to say, "And now I'm having contractions and I don't know what to do."

Instead she continued with her explanations.

"Queen Woo was the most powerful woman who married us, so I think I may have conceived on the night of the ceremony where she married us. She also gave us a strong fertility blessing."

She sighed heavily into the phone. "I just don't know what to do," she said.

"Well, let's start at the beginning," I said, sitting up in bed. "What month did you and your husband get married?"

"September," she answered.

I leaned back on my pillows and smiled into the phone. I was relieved that this wasn't an emergency. It was just an unusual call. We figured out her due date and made an appointment for her first prenatal visit.

She and her husband arrived a few weeks later at my office in an exquisite sports car. Our visit was long. Her husband, a research physician and internist, was developing a new technique for detecting and treating allergies. He described many alternative therapies such as Chinese medicine and acupuncture. Roberta was an artist and preferred to work in her studio sculpting and painting. She also was dedicated to the long process of soul searching and used various methods such as "rebirthing" and psychoanalysis to explore her world. I enjoyed our visit and looked forward to working with them. Little did I know that their delivery would be one of my hardest.

Roberta went into labor eight weeks early, after her bag of waters broke. She had been having some mild contractions before her bag of waters broke. I suggested consulting with my back-up doctor, but Ron, a physician himself, was convinced that the contractions would stop if Roberta drank alcohol and used some alternative remedies. Although her contractions slowed considerably, they resumed again when her bag of waters broke.

I was in the area doing some home visits when they called, so I went over to their home. Indeed, she was having contractions that were about ten minutes apart. I decided not to do a vaginal exam because I didn't want to expose her baby to possible infections. And I knew I was going to transfer her to the hospital soon anyway, and they would do a lot of vaginals.

When I called my consulting physician I discovered he was out of town for a few days. I had no backup. I called another doctor who was sympathetic to home births, but he was out of town also. Ron and Roberta were so far away from my other back-up doctors that the expecting parents refused to travel that far.

After numerous phone calls, I ventured back to tell them that I wanted them to go to the emergency room of the local hospital. It was the regional tertiary center for that part of the state, so it had an excellent neonatal intensive care unit for premature babies. While I was on the phone, however, Roberta and Ron came to some of their own decisions.

When I walked in, Ron was rubbing Roberta's back.

"How are the contractions doing?" I asked.

"They're about eight to ten minutes apart," Ron answered.

Roberta was on her hands and knees.

"I tried my best to contact my back-up physician, but he was gone and his back-up won't take people who have planned a homebirth. I also called a few other doctors and they are either out of town or won't work with us. I really think we ought to go to the emergency room as soon as we can."

Ron looked at me. "We've decided we don't want to go in," he said. He hurriedly went on. "Before you came I called around. I can get an oxygen tank with humidified oxygen and an incubator. I know a pediatrician who will come over and help us take care of the baby."

I really couldn't believe what I was hearing.

"You can't stay home," I said. "Premature babies really need the support of a neonatal intensive care unit. Plus, we don't know if the baby is okay. What if it's younger than we think it is? What if it has extra problems that would prevent it from breathing right away? It's a tremendous risk you're taking."

He seemed to waiver.

"Well, let me call my friend," he said.

He went to the phone. I tried to convince Roberta. She just looked at me and smiled a resigned smile. "Ron's a doctor," she said. "He knows what he's doing," she said quietly.

Ron came back into the room.

"My friend says we should stay at home," he said. Whereas he looked unsure before, he had a renewed sense of confidence.

"Is he willing to come here and manage this labor?" I asked.

Ron hesitated. "I'm sure he would come if I asked him."

"Go ahead and ask," I said.

He went to call again. After a few minutes I went to the phone.

"Let me talk to him," I said.

Ron gave me the phone.

After a short introduction, I vehemently stated my case.

"I'm surprised that you would encourage this couple to stay home and deliver this premature baby without any extra help from a neonatal intensive care unit," I stated.

"Oh, I think those units do more harm than good," he said.

"Well, I don't know if you're right or not, but I resent you advising them to stay at home and leaving me to deliver the baby. I think you ought to come here to manage the labor and take care of the baby if you're going to give that kind of advice," I said emphatically.

There was a pause on the other end of the line. "All right, I'll come right after I finish here at the office," he sighed. "If the baby is born before I arrive, don't cut the cord until you're sure the baby is breathing entirely on its own."

"When are you going to be finished with your office hours?" I asked.

"Within the hour," he answered.

"And, how long will it take you to drive here?" I asked.

"A little over an hour" was the answer.

"I think you should come right away," I said.

"I'll do the best I can" was his response.

I hung up the phone and went back to the bedroom to join Ron and Roberta.

"He said he would come," I told them.

"So, you'll stay with us?" Ron asked.

Amazingly, it hadn't crossed my mind to leave them. Legally, I knew I should to protect myself. This was a complicated delivery and out of the bounds of my protocols. None of my colleagues would stand in support of me if I was investigated for this. In fact, in the worst scenario, I could lose my license and be stripped of my certification. I should just pack my bag and walk out. But ethically, the story was entirely different. Even though Ron was a doctor, I knew that he knew nothing about delivering babies. I knew he wouldn't be able to resuscitate a premature infant. At least I had some experience in neonatal units and I had learned how to deliver premature babies in midwifery school. In short, the baby would have a greater chance of surviving if I stayed. There was no question in my mind of what I should do. I couldn't leave them. Nevertheless, I still tried to get them to go to the emergency room, especially because it looked like Roberta's labor had picked up and their pediatrician friend might not make it after all.

I decided to try a different tactic. Maybe I could call someone else in the alternative field—someone they respected—and get that person to help me convince them to go in. I knew exactly who to call.

"I'd like to call Irene Galbraith and ask her some questions about delivering premature babies," I said.

Irene was a direct entry midwife who had written a few books in the last few years. Roberta and Ron had her books, and I knew that they liked her philosophies. If anyone could convince them, she could.

I found her number and called her. Luckily she answered the phone. I explained my situation to her. She was wonderfully supportive of me. "It sounds like maybe I can help you," she said. "If my experience gives me the ability to help others, I'll be glad to talk to them. They need to go to the hospital and there's no question about it."

I called Ron to the phone.

"Irene wants to talk to you," I said.

I left him with the phone. I went back to Roberta to help her through her contractions. Things were looking serious. She was very self-absorbed. I knew it was useless to try again to talk to her about transferring. She had moved beyond communication. This baby was going to be born soon.

Ron came back into the room. He went up to Roberta and sat next to her.

"Hi," he whispered quietly to her. She smiled at him.

"I just talked to Irene," he started. "She agrees with Juliana and thinks we ought to go to the hospital." He hesitated for a moment while she concentrated through another contraction. "I think we should go in," he said to her. "We'll try to make it as easy as possible for you," he assured her. "And I'll fight to keep the baby with us."

I jumped at the opportunity.

"Good," I said. "Let's go now!"

I started to get her ready to go. It was hard to get her dressed between her contractions. I went as fast as I could. Ron did nothing to help. He paced back and forth in the room.

"I've got to make a phone call," he said as he suddenly rushed from the room.

"Good," I thought to myself. "He's going to call the rescue squad."

I continued to get Roberta ready.

Moments later Ron rushed into the room.

"I just called Dr. Madrison in New York," he said excitedly. "He agrees with me. He says we should keep Roberta at home. He says that the best place for premature babies to be born is at home."

My heart fell to my stomach.

"Oh no," I said. "You can't be serious about changing your plans. You need more professional help than I have to offer. You've got to transfer her to the hospital now!"

"No," he exclaimed emphatically. "I can help you. We've got everything we need here!" (The humidified oxygen he had ordered earlier in the day had arrived a few hours before.)

He rushed to Roberta's side. "Here I am," he said gently to her. "We're staying right here. I'll help you have this baby."

I was stunned. I numbly walked out of the room to gather my wits. I thought it was ironic that the midwives involved in this case wanted the mother to deliver in the hospital and the doctors wanted her to deliver at home. I gazed out of their living room window, hoping I would see their pediatrician friend pull up in the driveway. There was no one.

I heard a familiar grunting sound coming from the bedroom. Roberta was pushing. I rushed in. Her perineum was bulging with the impending delivery of the baby's head. I quickly listened to the heartbeat. Luckily it had seemed to be the only thing that stayed stable on this day. I heard it ticking away. I put on my gloves and cut an episiotomy. (It is the majority opinion that one should cut an episiotomy at the delivery of a premature baby so that the resistance of the mother's perineum doesn't cause injury to the baby's soft, underdeveloped cranium.)

The baby slid out into my hands. She was perfect. She was so tiny that I had no trouble holding her in one hand. She cried a weak perfunctory cry and then lay still. Ron, finally recognizing the seriousness of the situation, called the rescue squad.

I started working on her. I put her on Roberta's abdomen and started suctioning and resuscitating her. She lay still. I checked her heart rate. It was present, going about 120 beats per minute. She seemed to respond to my oxygen administration, but she couldn't breathe on her own. After a few minutes, she pinked up. But I continued my resuscitation efforts. I was afraid to stop. I heard the sirens as the rescue squad approached. The whole episode is punctuated in my mind by the blowing of the oxygen tank, the sirens and the commotion as the squad entered the living room. All of the commotion seemed to surround me as I was pulled into the vacuum of the baby's stillness and Roberta's stillness as she watched me working on the baby on her abdomen.

Suddenly everyone rushed into the bedroom. Their friend, the pediatrician, arrived at the same time.

His voice took command. "Wait out in the living room," he ordered the rescue squad. "I will get the baby stabilized for transport."

They obeyed him and left the room.

He walked over to us on the bed. The baby was quite pink and crying now. She was alive! Her tiny limbs were waving in the air! Her eyes were opened! I stayed next to her as if I was guarding her. I was ready to start on her again if she showed me any sign that she was faltering. She didn't.

The pediatrician finally picked her up. She was crying in his arms. He checked her over. I watched numbly.

She looked so good. She seemed to be holding her own quite well. How strong life is!

He grunted his approval and took her out to the rescue squad. Soon, the sirens faded into the evening sunset.

I left Roberta and Ron's house in a daze. I left Roberta tucked in bed, with a friend who had come to take care of her. Ron had followed the baby to the hospital.

I was angry when I got home. How could they have done this? How could they have endangered the life of their tiny daughter? I spent the evening ranting and raving about it. I also learned another lesson: When I was in another person's house, I was not in control.

I slept fitfully that night. I couldn't calm my mind. By morning I started my office hours with heavy eyes and a heavy heart. I was worried about the baby. I hoped that Ron would give me a call to update me on her status. I tried to keep my mind on my appointments.

Finally Ron called. He sounded excited.

"The baby's doing fine," he reported. "She weighs three pounds. She's in an incubator now and they have her on medications and oxygen. I've been talking to my colleagues, and I think that I might be able to bring her home in an incubator and care for her there."

"What do you mean?" I asked.

"Well, I really want her out of here. They are X-raying her constantly and then they wouldn't let me protect her incubator from the radiation scatter when they were X-raying other babies."

He went on. "I couldn't believe that they asked me to leave the room while the babies were being X-rayed," he said. "When I asked them why, they said because of the danger of the radiation scatter. I said then that I wanted to stand in front of the incubator so that my baby would be protected. That's why I want her out of here. There are so many things going on here that aren't to her benefit."

He continued telling me about the neonatal intensive care unit (NICU) and all of its hazards. Roberta was with the baby now, and they were trying to stay with her around the clock so that she would have a sense of security from their presence. They also had already asked their religious leader to come in and bless the baby. We finished our conversation with the promise to keep in daily contact.

The next day Ron called with the news that they were well on their way to being able to bring the baby home. They had found a few neonatal nurses who were willing to work for them around the clock on shifts. He was negotiating their salaries with them. He had also secured an incubator from a company in another state. He was presently negotiating with a pediatrician to come to the home once a day to supervise the care. His friend who arrived at the birth would consult by phone.

The following day Ron called with the good news that he had secured commitments from the neonatal nurses, and the pediatrician had also agreed. All plans were in force and they were going to take the baby out the next day when the incubator arrived. Meanwhile the baby was doing well. Ron was especially anxious to get her home because Roberta was getting exhausted staying with the baby and expressing milk from her breasts to feed her through a nasogastric tube.

On the third day, the bomb dropped on their plans. The chief physician at the NICU heard about what they intended to do. It angered him and his attack was fast and furious. He threatened the NICU nurses with their jobs if they worked in Ron's arrangement. He called the pediatrician and guaranteed that the hospital would not receive any of his patients nor make new patient referrals to him if he worked with Ron. He called the incubator company and encouraged them to postpone delivery. And, worst of all, he threatened to get a judge to strip Ron and Roberta of their parental rights and claim that the baby was a "ward of the state" if they insisted on removing the baby from the premises. He even called the Board of Medicine in an attempt to strip Ron of his medical license.

Ron and Roberta stayed with their baby for two more weeks in the hospital. They were tired and haggard. Roberta continued to express milk. They continued their vigil. They continued to protect her against the radiation scatter. They covered her incubator at night so she would have a break from the constant lighting. They put a tape of Roberta's heartbeat next to her. They laid her on a soft sheepskin in the incubator. And they continued to get blessings from their religious leaders.

They called me regularly and I cheered them on. My anger had long ago turned into admiration. Their experience opened up a whole new set of questions for me. What about all of these interventions done in the NICU? Are we harming babies while we're helping them? What happens to the families of these babies? Ron and Roberta were exhausted from their efforts. There was no place for Roberta to lie down as she stayed with her little one. And, in her increasing fatigue, she had a harder and harder time expressing her breastmilk. She also claimed that the overload of beeps, buzzing, and lights made it difficult for her to rest in her chair. She wondered how much actual rest her baby was getting. Ron was driving back and forth from home to hospital in a continual state of preoccupation and fatigue. It's a small wonder he never got in a car accident. The immense stress on Ron and Roberta made me worry about those families who had no money and no home, or who lived far away from the NICUs. How did they make it? Or, did they make it? Is it any surprise that premature babies are the most likely to be neglected or abused? Disaster surrounds their births, they're separated from their families for prolonged periods and finally, when they are reunited, the parents feel totally inept to perform the frustrating job of parenting them.

Concurrently however, other questions of ethics were raised. Can our system take all the parental rights away from parents if one doctor believes that the parents are not acting in the best interests of the child? It was frightening how quickly Ron and Roberta's child could be taken away from them. This experience only solidified in Ron and Roberta's minds that they were right: They probably shouldn't have taken the baby to the hospital in the first place. Are more people going to react that way? Are more people going to perceive the hospital as their enemy and therefore not go to it in times of trouble? Yes, Ron and Roberta are of the alternative mind set, the ones who travel the roads that no one else does, but maybe we should look at their example and prevent their situation from happening to us "more normal" folks.

It was in the fall of 1985 that CNMs were dropped by our liability insurance carrier. Because of a liability insurance crisis across the country, everyone was getting hit hard by the "soft" investment market. (Insurance companies invest premiums in high-interest markets so that they can make a lot of money on their income. A soft market meant that interest rates were plunging and they were not able to make very much money on their investments.) At the same time, there was a lot of hysteria about suing. Obstetricians were getting sued frequently and for high amounts.

I've always had a theory about the malpractice crisis. I think malpractice is a rudimentary form of regulation. The reason why it has hit physicians so hard is because they aren't adequately regulated. They may think they are adequately regulated, and they complain bitterly about the many restrictions against their practice, but for years they have regulated themselves through a good old boy network. In this protective framework, private physicians can pretty much treat health problems however they want to. If they want to treat a woman's temporary nervousness with Valium, they can. If they want to do a hysterectomy for benign growths on the uterus, they can. If they want to do a cesarean for a normal breech presentation, they can. Physicians have always been deferred to as the experts.

However, people have suffered and paid too much for the physician's actions because often those actions have been financially motivated. This is especially true in obstetrics. Obstetricians can use all sorts of technology to control a birth. They can induce a woman to deliver her baby on a day when their appointments and surgeries aren't heavy. They can artificially stimulate a labor so it doesn't interfere with other plans. They can sedate a woman so that she doesn't go into active labor in the middle of the night. And, in borderline cases, why not do a cesarean instead of waiting for potential fetal distress and resulting lawsuit? No wonder obstetric health care costs have reached astronomical levels.

Unfortunately, we are beginning to find out that all of these interventions beget trouble. The uterus is not a muscle to be toyed with. Obstetricians forcing a normal uterus to contract at the pace and intensity they want is as ludicrous as cardiologists forcing a normal heart to beat at the pace and velocity they want.

By having the power to regulate how, when and where a woman delivers her baby, obstetricians place themselves as the ultimate decision makers. So, if something goes wrong, the family blames the obstetrician. This blame is accentuated by the anger and helplessness that is felt during the normal grieving process. To add insult to injury, the obstetrician rarely takes the time to explain what happened to the patient nor do they encourage open communication between themselves and the patient.

The ACNM was up in arms about this insurance crisis. Although CNMs rarely got sued (6 percent versus the obstetricians' 60 percent), we were perceived by the insurance companies as just as high risk because we worked in the same field. Because our coverage would be higher than our salaries, we lost the coverage. Many nurse-midwifery services and birthing centers closed. It was almost impossible to find an insurance company who would cover us.

ACNM started looking into self-insurance. The members would pay premiums to the ACNM and they would cover us. Suddenly, a consortium of liability companies offered insurance to us. ACNM jumped at the consortium's plan and accepted the coverage.

The original crisis of not having insurance was over, only to be replaced by the crisis of having very expensive premiums. Basically, our liability insurance jumped from costing less than $200 a year to more that $2500 a year. We would also have to purchase a "tail." Because in obstetrics we can get sued until the baby is eleven years old, a "tail" allows us to retain our coverage for eleven years to cover ourselves for a baby we delivered today.

During this crisis, I made some decisions. I carried malpractice insurance before, but now I didn't know if I wanted to pay the exorbitant price for the premiums. I would have to pass the cost over to my clients. The initial reason for liability insurance is to protect a patient from financial ruin as a result of damages caused by a health care provider's neglect. But I don't neglect people and I communicate to them that they are responsible for taking care of themselves. I am their consultant and advisor. My responsibility is teaching, screening and assessment. Their responsibility is to care. I believe that the more time you spend with someone and the more respectfully you treat them, the less likely they are to sue. With that in mind, I canceled my insurance and started practicing without it. I know, however, that I'm not immune from liability, so I have transferred everything I own over to Eric. I always told my clients my liability situation so, if they were uncomfortable with my philosophy, they could leave my service.

In September of 1985 I started volunteering prenatal care in a local migrant health clinic. I also offered free prenatal classes at a local church. The job at the migrant health clinic didn't last too long because as soon as the malpractice crisis hit, they couldn't work with me anymore. That was unfortunate because at the same time the local obstetricians refused prenatal services to all uninsured women unless the woman could pay $900 at her first prenatal visit. Most women couldn't afford this so they put off their first visit until it was too late. Many women were forced to go without care or go to the nurse clinic at the public health department.

When I found out about this I called the director of the public health department to offer my services for prenatal care. Despite my numerous offers, he turned them down. It seemed that he would rather the women receive no prenatal care than risk the wrath of the local obstetricians who insisted that I work under the direct supervision of a physician. I was frustrated that the nurses at the public health department (who had no extra training in this specialty) could provide prenatal care without physician supervision, but I, who was an expert in the field, couldn't work without a physician directly supervising me. No, the director wouldn't hire me but he did concede to let the nurses use a grant from the March of Dimes to pay me to teach them how to provide the care.

The rest of my year was spent peacefully delivering babies. Jodie was a 19-year-old woman having her first baby. She came to me for the first time when she was six months pregnant. She had not had any prenatal care, and she was seeking my care because I was less expensive than the doctors and she was afraid to go to the hospital. She was a hairdresser and lived with her boyfriend, Jeff, and some other roommates. She was anemic but wasn't on any iron supplements and was only taking one multivitamin a day. Her pregnancy was unplanned.

Jodie started under my care when I was still doing home visits for the first visit. When I arrived at Jodie's house, I found her to be a shy woman who was unsure about having a midwife and home delivery but really was stuck in the reality of having no money to go elsewhere. She knew she didn't want to go to the clinic because she did once and "didn't receive any care." Throughout the visit, the TV was on as background noise. There were pictures of rock stars on the walls. I reminded myself that if I had been a teenager, my house would have looked much the same.

Jodie wore a lot of make-up and her nails were long and red. Her hair was made up in a meticulous hairstyle. Upon finding out that she was a hairdresser, I fought back the temptation to ask her what I should do with my hair.

Jeff, Jodie's boyfriend, arrived in the middle of my three-hour visit and stayed around to listen to all I had to say. I think he was slightly overwhelmed at the depth I went into when I introduced them to my service.

While I asked her all the questions that I usually ask at my first visit (past medical history, family history, and so forth), I wondered how I was going to get a healthy baby out of this woman. She was a heavy soda drinker and didn't look like she spent much time thinking about her diet. I immediately told her to cut out all of her sodas and as I always do, I told her to give me a three-day diet history at her next visit, which I scheduled for two weeks later.

By Jodie's third visit, things were really shaping up. She had started noticing a decrease in fatigue and leg cramps. She stopped drinking 10 percent juice and switched to 100 percent. She stopped all of her caffeine sodas and only had one decaf soda a week. She was putting wheat germ in her homemade burgers and on cereal. She even found that the nonfat dry milk powder I had told her to add to her milk wasn't so bad, and because she was concerned about excess weight gain, she was pleased that she could pull all this extra protein into her diet without adding extra fat. Jeff and I were both really proud of her. Jeff even stopped taking her to fast food restaurants and enjoyed the financial savings.

After nine more prenatal visits and my continual nagging, Jodie was good and ready to go into labor. She called me in the morning at 6:45 A.M. to tell me that she had been having contractions since 3:00 A.M. and now they were fifteen to twenty minutes apart. She even had some bloody show, but her bag of waters wasn't broken yet. We joked a little bit and Jeff got on the phone to brush up on last minute instructions: get plenty of rest, drink plenty of water and juices, call me if any danger signs appear (quick review of the signs included), and call me when you want me to come.

When she called back at 9:00 A.M. she said there was no change in her contractions but I sensed a little anxiety in her voice so I decided to go to her house to calm things down. I arrived at 11:00 A.M. and the contractions were now five to ten minutes apart. The baby's heartbeat sounded good and Jodie's blood pressure was normal.

We spent the day doing various things. We watched TV. I sent her and Jeff for a nap in the afternoon. She rested well and at 3:30 P.M. she was six to seven centimeters dilated.

By evening, some of her friends brought over a pizza so my birth assistant and I joined Jeff and his friends for dinner. Jodie didn't feel much like eating, so I kept her nourished with yogurt, Gatorade, Jell-O and soups. I made sure that something passed through her mouth every fifteen minutes.

By 8:00 P.M. her contractions were really coming strong. They were about three to five minutes apart, and she was eight to nine centimeters dilated.

The house had taken on a quieter, more serious tone. All of her friends had gone home. Jodie took a shower for about ten minutes, and we walked around the house. During contractions, she squatted while leaning against her couch. She especially liked this during the harder contractions. When she got tired, she rested on her side. I listened to her baby's heartbeat every 15 minutes and it sounded great.

Jeff was a great help. She leaned on him a lot and he supported her while she squatted. He broke out in a sweat a few times. I remained watchful.

By about 8:30 P.M. she was getting pretty fed up with everything and I decided that we probably needed a change of atmosphere. It was a beautiful evening and the stars were out, so why not walk outside for a while? I bundled her up (it was late fall) and we drove to a nice secluded country road. I parked the car in the driveway of one of my previous clients and we walked under the full moon for over an hour. She leaned on Jeff's arm and squatted with the contractions. I carried the juice and the flashlight. Every ten minutes we stopped so I could listen to the baby's heartbeat while she stood still. I even listened to it through the contractions a few times. While we walked we talked about Jeff's job, Jodie's hairdressing job, and their plans for the baby. It was fun.

At about 10:30 P.M. Jodie started to feel an urge to push with her contractions so we slowly walked back to the car and drove home. I checked her at 11:00 P.M. and she was fully dilated and ready to push.

After 47 minutes of pushing in both the sidelying position and the squatting position, their beautiful baby girl was born at 11:47 P.M. The baby's hand was born together with her head, but we didn't have any perineal tears. Jodie stayed very controlled so we could deliver the head slowly and smoothly. The baby was beautifully pink and ready to get to know everyone. Jodie nursed her immediately, which helped reduce the uterine bleeding. She didn't lose much blood and my job developed into one of just watching a beautiful process take place.

Thanksgiving day was spent at a long birth. Sandra was a wonderful woman who loves children and loves being pregnant, but I came away from this labor convinced that some women just have their babies hard.

This was Sandra's second baby. Her first was delivered by direct entry midwives in California. She called me early in the morning and I arrived to find her contractions far apart but strong. I encouraged her to alternate resting and walking because I knew she had a long way to go. I stayed with her all day, only leaving for a short while to have Thanksgiving dinner next door at her brother's home.

After dinner I came back to find that her labor really hadn't changed much. I felt the position of the baby and discovered, to my dismay, that it had turned to the posterior position. It was a big baby, so I knew that Sandra's day was going to be long. We tried a variety of positions. I had her on her hands and knees. We tried squatting. She rested on her side. I watched her get more and more fatigued, but her spirits were unquenchable. She just kept encouraging her baby. She would keep rubbing her belly and talking to her baby. "Come on, little one," she would say. "I know that we can do it together. Don't you worry, when you come out, Mama's going to give you lots of hugs and warm milk."

The afternoon turned into evening and the evening into night. The hours wore on. Her contractions started fizzling out. They were not as strong as before. I was worried. I knew she was wearing down. Her uterus just wasn't turning this baby around and pushing it down.

The walls of their little home seemed to cave in on us. Jim, Sandra's husband, was looking ragged. He had supported Sandra for the past eighteen hours. He didn't want to leave her side. Earlier in the evening I had sent him next door to get some Thanksgiving dinner, but he gobbled it up quickly and came rushing back. Now he was sustaining himself on coffee.

I was getting weary myself. I started to wonder if I should transfer her and hook her up to pitocin by IV to stimulate her contractions. All she needed was strong contractions to turn the baby and push it out. I hesitated discussing this option with them. I knew them well. They were very committed to having their baby without intervention and because the baby showed no signs of distress, they would not want to go in.

Suddenly I had another idea. I looked at Sandra and Jim on the bed.

"Let's go out for a ride," I said to them.

They turned to look at me. Their eyes were blank.

"Let's get in your Scout and drive through the national park," I continued. "I'll bring my fetoscope to listen to the baby and maybe the bumpy ride will help you out. Besides, the change of scenery might help you."

Of course, the scenery would amount to nothing. It was a dark and misty night.

Jim agreed. I helped Sandra struggle into her clothes and she lumbered out to the car.

Jim drove and my birth assistant sat up front with him. Sandra and I sat in the back. We started down the road.

I had another idea.

"Now," I said to Sandra, "I'm going to do something strange. I'm going to twist your nipples with my fingers to stimulate you to have contractions. You can lean on me and rest. We're going to try to get a lot of strong contractions. I hope that, together with this drive, we might be able to get this baby out."

I put my arm around her and reached up under her sweater and started twisting her nipples. She leaned her head on my shoulder.

It felt strange to me to be in this position with another woman. I couldn't believe that my life had come to this. Here I was, sitting in a truck twiddling a woman's nipples in Shenandoah National Park in the middle of the night.

"Gee, Juliana," I thought to myself, "you have to write a book."

We drove around for quite awhile. Suddenly, her contractions started coming closer together. First they were every five minutes, then every three minutes, then every two minutes. She started to have to breathe heavily through them.

We had quite a system going. I would twiddle her nipples until she started a contraction. She would signal a contraction coming with a soft "Now." When it was over she would say "okay." I would listen to the baby and then I would start on her nipples again.

She started to feel more vaginal pressure. It was increasing! Jim turned the car around and started home.

When we arrived, she started to feel like she had to push. We held her in a squatting position. I could feel the baby coming down. Jim continued the nipple stimulation. We could see the top of the baby's head at the opening of her vagina.

There was renewed energy in the room. We were cheering her on. Sandra seemed to have a spurt of adrenalin. "C'mon baby," she kept saying. "Come on out and see your Mama!"

Finally their little boy was born. He was ten pounds and four ounces. He was beautiful. We all collapsed together in happy exhaustion. He suckled immediately while we watched in awe.

10

IN 1986 one of my deliveries started me on a tumultuous political path that was the most significant threat to my personal and professional existence.

Marie was a 29-year-old woman having her fourth baby. They were a simple family with not much money but a lot of faith in their religion. Marie's older children were schooled at home as her husband tried desperately to make ends meet operating a solo house painting business. They contacted me to help them have their baby at home for financial reasons. They just couldn't afford the rising cost of health care.

Marie was a quiet woman and very sweet. We got along well together and she followed my directions faithfully. Her pregnancy progressed normally, but her past pregnancy history was a little worrisome. About two weeks after the birth of her last child she bled too much. She was convinced it was because the doctor had pulled so hard on the placenta before it was ready to come that some placenta fragments had stayed behind. And, with one of her earlier babies, she bled excessively in the recovery room two hours after the birth. But her bladder had been full because they'd left her alone for so long after the delivery, and she couldn't get up to go to the bathroom. A full bladder can cause a woman to hemorrhage because it can prevent the uterus from contracting and closing up. Only after the nurses catheterized her bladder did she finally stop bleeding.

During her present pregnancy I detected a growth on her uterus called a fibroid, but after a sonogram, my consulting physician and I felt it wouldn't be a problem.

"What about the problems with postpartum bleeding that she had with two of her previous pregnancies?" I asked Dr. Call.

"Juliana," he answered. "You know that both of these were caused by intervention performed at the hospital. She'll be okay."

I agreed with him. Because so many hemorrhages are caused by intervention, I was far less suspicious of a hemorrhage that occurred in the hospital than I was of those that occurred at home with midwives. Those worry me and I might consider a woman with a hemorrhage at a previous home birth too risky for a home birth again.

Marie called me one day in early spring. She was in labor. Her contractions were severe so I went to her home right away. We called her birth assistant, a nurse I didn't know. Marie delivered her baby girl beautifully, but after the birth of the placenta, she began acting restless. She just wouldn't focus on the baby, and she was pale, clammy, and nauseated. Her uterus felt contracted and there was hardly any bleeding, but I knew something was wrong. Women don't act this way after birth and I have long since learned that if a mother shows a lack of interest in her baby, something is not right.

I decided to check her vulvar area. Maybe there was a clot that was blocking her blood flow. Sure enough, I found one. It was like a dam. I braced myself and pulled it out. It was the size of a tangerine. Suddenly the blood started gushing out of her vagina. It was as if someone had turned on the faucet. I put my hand in her vagina to grab her uterus from the inside and put my other hand on her abdomen to grab her uterus on the outside. I massaged the uterus vigorously between both hands to help it contract. I instructed my birth assistant to call the rescue squad and administer my emergency medications to help her uterus to contract.

We started an IV. The rescue squad came. The bleeding had slowed down considerably and I called my consulting physician.

"If you have it under control, stay there and give her some more methergine." (Methergine is a medication that helps the uterus contract.) He continued, "If you're worried, come in."

The rescue squad was waiting for my decision.

"I just talked to my consulting physician and I'd like to wait a few moments to see if she remains under control," I explained to them.

"Who's the doc, ma'am?" the man asked.

I told him.

"Never heard of him. Is he new here?" he asked.

I explained that he worked out of a hospital close by but not in this community.

"We can't take her there, ma'am," he said. "We have to take her to this hospital."

"Oh no," I thought to myself. "That means she'll have to go to the doctor on call. He won't know her and maybe will admonish her for having a home birth. Besides, the hospital bill will be enormous."

"We'll stay here," I decided.

The rescue squad left.

I checked her bleeding and blood pressure. They were both normal. She was becoming more responsive to her baby. I was breathing a little easier, but I still kept an eye on her.

Suddenly she started bleeding again. We gave her more medication. She stopped bleeding. I was feeling unsure. She had lost a lot of blood by now and even though she'd stopped bleeding, I knew she might again and again.

I decided to call the rescue squad again. An exasperated crew returned and put her in the ambulance. I followed them to the hospital. It was 12:00 midnight.

We went straight up to labor and delivery. The doctor on call was Dr. Gordon, an obstetrician. He gave orders to the nurse on duty by phone. Basically we had already done everything that he ordered. We had already put in an IV, we had already given the medications he ordered and we were already monitoring her blood pressure and pulse frequently.

"Just watch her, then," he instructed.

The nurse got busy and we were left alone. The clock ticked away. The hours passed. The doctor neither called nor showed up. I kept monitoring her bleeding, blood pressure and pulse. She had no more episodes of increased bleeding. Her older daughter, husband and friend kept the baby out in the hallway.

About two hours went by before it dawned on me that we were doing the same thing that we would have done at home. The only difference was the building. The doctor on call was at home and could be contacted by phone just as my own consulting physician could. I was amazed that the doctor didn't even bother to show up. He just let the nurses manage her and they weren't even in the room. They came in periodically to report the blood pressures that I took. What kind of emergency care was this?

I stayed with her until 4:00 A.M. She was stable and waiting for the doctor to discharge her. I rushed home to get ready for office hours.

I was flabbergasted by this experience. I just transferred a woman to the hospital and performed all of her care myself. I should have kept them at home. Now this financially strapped couple would have a huge hospital bill for nothing.

Later that morning Marie called me. They were home. Dr. Gordon had arrived at 8:00 A.M. He admonished her for having a home birth. He fiercely massaged her uterus and barked his discharge orders to the nurse and left.

A few days later Karen, a nurse-midwife who worked as a nurse at the hospital I transferred to, phoned me.

"Dr. Gordon is furious about the transfer you made the other night," she said. "He insists that she was high-risk for a home birth and you should never have attempted it."

"What makes him think that she was high risk?" I asked.

"She had two previous hemorrhages and she has that growth on her uterus.

Really Juliana, you have to learn to say no to some of the people who call you," she warned.

"Karen, I say no to so many people," I sighed into the phone. "I won't take smokers or women who are overweight, or women who have had previous hemorrhages. But Marie was different."

I explained Marie's history to Karen. She agreed with me that her previous hemorrhages sounded like they were hospital induced.

"Well, Dr. Gordon is not going to be convinced," she said. "He's threatening to report you to the Board of Health."

"Give him my number and have him call me," I said. "I'll explain this to him and then he can do what he wants. But, I'm at peace with myself that I made the right decision."

A few days later he called. His words gushed into the phone.

"I'm calling the Board of Health on you," he screamed. "I think what you're doing is illegal. I'm going to find out the rules about home birth. I bet you're breaking them!"

I waited for him to calm down.

"I work closely with many members on the regulatory boards," I explained quietly. "I can assure you that I have not done anything illegal."

I explained to him the guidelines under which I practice.

"Who's your supervising physician?" he asked. "Why didn't you take her to him?"

I explained that the rescue squad wouldn't transfer Marie to my back-up hospital.

"Well, I don't appreciate being involved in this business. I'll make sure you don't practice anymore."

"You have to do what you have to do," I said to him. I refused to beg him or apologize to him.

He slammed the phone on the hook.

I stared out the window. My mind was blank and my body was trembling.

A few weeks later I received a call from an investigator from the Board of Health regarding a complaint that Dr. Gordon had filed against me. He questioned me about the case. I sent in the chart. A committee from the Board would review it and send a recommendation to the Board.

Dr. Call was extremely supportive.

"Don't worry, Juliana," he assured me. "They just want to harass you. I'll stick behind you."

He laughed into the phone. "We should just start filing complaints about some of these jokers and the way they practice. A lot of them would be out of business!"

The investigator called Dr. Call, and he went through an hour of questioning. He called me when the investigator left.

"Really, Juliana, the only thing that went wrong here is that I should have called the hospital and warned them you were coming in."

The months went by and I heard nothing else. I realized for the first time how slowly the system worked. Absolutely nothing was going on. I didn't know whether that was a bad sign.

In the spring I attended one of the quarterly meetings of a board appointed by the governor to recommend changes in the state's maternity health care system. It was held in Richmond, and I went because I'd heard through the grapevine that the subject of midwifery would be discussed.

The board was composed largely of physicians, and three of the OB/GYNs on the board were known to be enemies of midwives. I took a seat behind one the of the OB/GYNs who was sitting at the board table.

A doctor began the meeting by asking, "What are we going to do with the midwives?"

"Certified nurse-midwives have decreased the infant mortality rate in every area where they practice," one board member said. "We've got to find a way to use them in the system."

"We don't want them practicing independently," a physician countered. "If we let that happen, all hell will break loose!"

Then the doctor in front of me started talking. "I don't mind midwives," he said. "Why, I have a friend who uses a midwife in his office. He really likes her. She does the simple things so he can concentrate on more important matters." I cringed at the insinuation that we could be used by doctors to do the work they didn't think was worth their while.

"But by God, we've got to watch these midwives who go out there and practice all by themselves." He threw a pile of papers down on the table. "Why, I've got a whole mess of studies here from all over the nation that say that midwives are dangerous! I also have a letter here that an OB/GYN sent to the Board of Health about a nurse-midwife in the Winchester area who dumped a lady hemorrhaging after a home birth, leaving him to save her life!"

My spine crawled. My face was burning.

"That's me he's talking about," I thought to myself.

The nurse-midwife with me glanced at me. I tried to see the letter the doctor was waving about. I couldn't see it.

My thoughts were racing.

"How could the story get distorted like that?" I thought. "How am I going to clear my reputation with these people?"

I felt sick to my stomach with desperation. I wished I could run away from all this to the security of my home, children, and Eric. I didn't want to fight anymore.

Suddenly I thought of something. The laws about investigations came back to me. The investigator had referred to them when he'd spoken to me. My case was supposed to be kept confidential until a decision was made. Only when the decision is made does it become public record. How did this doctor, who isn't even on the Board of Health, get this letter? How did he even know about my case?

My growing anger gave me energy. "I'm going to get to the bottom of this and, by golly, if my head rolls, so will a few others!"

The Chairman of the Board called for a break. I jumped up and went to the doctor.

"Pardon me," I said. "I'm interested in seeing those studies about the dangers of midwifery practice." I pointed to the stack of papers he had thrown on the table.

He looked slightly embarrassed. I could tell he wasn't used to being held accountable for his words.

"Oh, those are just a pile of laws regarding midwifery practice all over the United States," he said.

"Oh, I must be mistaken," I said. "I thought they were studies about the dangers of midwifery practice."

"No, no," he said, waving the papers aside. "But, this case about the midwife out there doing home births and dumping hemorrhages on the doctors needs to be looked into." His temporary embarrassment gave way to bluster.

I tried to read as much of the letter as I could without looking too interested. I saw that it was from Dr. Gordon and addressed to the Board of Health. I saw my name in the text. It wasn't the original, but it did have an official looking stamp on it noting that it had been received by the Board. But before I could discover more, the break was over and I went back to my chair.

The next morning, I called Carla Darsh, one of the officials of the Board. She liked me and was glad that I was working on the state level in support of midwifery. In fact, she considered me the expert on midwifery in the state.

"Hi, Juliana," she said into the phone. "What can I do for you?"

I explained what had happened the day before. I had a copy of the Code of Virginia in front of me.

"I'm sure that something illegal has happened, Carla," I said to her. "My case is supposed to be confidential and here it was broadcast all over the room at this meeting! Not only was it broadcast, but it was exaggerated beyond belief. That man had the nerve to say that the doctor saved the woman's life when the actual truth was that he didn't even show up until eight hours after I transferred the patient. I managed her alone for the first four hours!"

"I can understand how you feel," she said. "But I have no idea how this happened."

"Well, I intend to find out," I insisted. "My next step is to call the Director of the Board of Health. I've got to pursue this, Carla. I can't let this pass, not only for my sake, but for the future of midwifery in this state!"

I hung up the phone. I sounded much more resolved than I actually felt. I was trembling again.

I decided to give myself a few days to calm down. The end of the week went by and the weekend passed. I calmed down and by Sunday I built up my resolve to make the next phone call.

A month later the letter came. It was from the Board of Nursing.

They had thoroughly investigated the complaint filed against me. They found no evidence to support the allegations; therefore, my record was cleared of any charges. The case was closed.

You would think that would have been the end of it. No such luck. Once a decision has been made by the Board regarding a case like mine, it becomes public record and any other Board can act on it if they want. Well, the Board of Medicine got a hold of it and they decided to go after my supervising physician.

One day an investigator from the Board of Medicine knocked on my door. He flashed his ID card as he introduced himself on my doorstep.

"May I come in?" he asked.

I stood back and let him in. I was shocked. What happened? What was wrong now?

Eric came into the room. The investigator introduced himself and we sat down.

"I'd like to know anything you might be able to tell me about Dr. Call," he began.

"Tell me why you are interested," I said.

"The Board of Medicine is investigating Dr. Call for his involvement in the case that was just decided in your favor," he informed me.

I couldn't believe my ears. It seemed that the medical profession wouldn't stop harassing me. Even though I delivered only four babies a month, they saw me as a threat to their existence. If they allowed me to go on, others would follow and people would see that midwives provide personalized quality care.

I stared at him silently. Eric, though, had had enough.

"That's despicable," he exclaimed. "And, you know, I also find it despicable that you came here to our home without making a prior appointment to talk with us! You drove all the way from Richmond to question Juliana. You should have called first. I don't appreciate you barging in here."

Eric got up from the couch and walked to the front door. The investigator fumbled with his papers and stood up.

"I was coming here on another matter and just decided to drop by," he murmured.

"You did, did you?" Eric persisted. "Well, I think you'd better go. The Board of Medicine is harassing midwives and the doctors who work with them. We will not tolerate it."

He slammed the door behind the investigator.

"There," he said triumphantly. "We won't see him again."

"Maybe not," I warned. "But the Board of Medicine is going to persist. They want to see me out of practice. I know I'll lose Dr. Call's support now. What do I do?"

I felt frightened and desperate. We'd have to move. I'd have to look for another job. I went to the phone. "I need to warn Dr. Call that he's coming."

I got Dr. Call's answering service. I didn't leave a message. I wanted to talk to him personally.

I continued to see patients that afternoon. In the early evening the phone rang. It was Dr. Call.

"Juliana," his voice boomed into the phone. "I had an interesting visitor this afternoon."

"I know," I said. "He came to see me too."

"Well, I told him in no uncertain terms that I considered this harassment, and if the Board of Medicine persisted in this underhanded manner that I would file some complaints against some of the Board members that would make their heads spin! Then I politely showed him the way out."

I told him what Eric did.

He laughed. "Poor guy. He had a bad day! I don't think we'll hear from him again!"

Relief washed over me. Dr. Call had his feet on the ground. He was sure of himself and was not going to be intimidated. There should be more people like him in this world. Someday I would be like that. But for now I shuddered at the thought of how close I was to losing my license. The doctors were ruthless and I was helpless. The only thing I had going for me was Dr. Call's support. I was vulnerable, but I became determined to fight for my rights.

We never heard from the Board of Medicine again . . . about this case.

Unfortunately, this wasn't the only event that made 1986 a tumultuous year. Another birth created another nightmare in my life.

Victor and Donna were a newlywed couple who came to me during her first pregnancy. She was a nurse and he was a surveyor. Their unplanned pregnancy had forced them to marry. They were very much in love, but I could tell that things were moving a little too fast for both of them. Nevertheless, they both had a ready sense of humor and we laughed a lot during our visits. Donna was also very kind and loving.

The arrangement for Donna's consulting physician was unusual. Donna lived on a farm in a beautiful mountainous area that was about an hour and a half from my supervising physician. Consequently, she visited an OB/GYN that was in the town close to her. He was very friendly and agreed to be available for consultation or to meet us in the hospital if necessary. My conversation with him went smoothly so I felt confident that we had a solid back-up arrangement.

Donna's pregnancy went well until the delivery. She rested a lot the week before she entered labor so she was in good shape. In fact, when I arrived, she looked radiant. Her contractions were strong and close together. She was progressing well.

We had a nice evening together. Things got rough for her, but she responded well to the love and support that was around her. She and Victor took a long bath together. Her contractions got stronger.

The phone rang at midnight. Another one of my patients, Debra, was in labor. Her contractions were five minutes apart and strong. I was in the dilemma that I always had nightmares about; two people in labor at the same time. I called Ann, a retired British-trained nurse-midwife. I was in luck. She agreed to go to Debra.

By early morning Donna's contractions were so strong that she had an urge to push. Her bag of waters broke. I was encouraged. I did a vaginal exam to feel if her cervix was completely dilated. There was still some cervix there and I felt that the baby had turned posterior. I also felt that the head wasn't well applied to the cervix. That means that the cervix, the opening of the uterus that the baby comes out of, wasn't fitting around the head very well.

Because her urge to push was so strong and almost impossible to stop, I let her push and I tried to hold the cervix out of the way. This is similar to using a shoe horn to fit a foot into a shoe. We tried that for a while but it didn't work. I knew that it wasn't good for her to push when the cervix was there because the baby's head would just cause the cervix to swell. Then it would really have a hard time opening up to let the baby through.

We tried everything. I put her in a variety of positions to try to stop her urge to push, and when that didn't work I again tried to hold the cervix back while she pushed. Finally it stayed back but the baby wasn't coming down at all. It was stuck. We needed help. Two hours of pushing with no progress was enough.

I called the hospital. A nurse answered the phone.

"This is Juliana Fehr. I'm a certified nurse-midwife. My patient, Donna Delaney, is in labor with second stage arrest (no progress once the mother starts pushing). Dr. Michaels is her consulting physician and I'm transferring her to his care."

"Dr. Michaels is on vacation so I'll give Dr. Gaynor, his partner, a call to tell him you are coming," she said. We put Donna in the back of my car and Victor sat next to her while I drove in.

The early morning was clear and dark. The country road seemed to wind endlessly. There was an unnerving quiet around me. The countryside was so pervasive that it seemed to echo the roar of my car's engine. It was like driving through a wide hollow tunnel of trees.

At the hospital Donna was wheeled to labor and delivery. An older nurse admitted her. She barely acknowledged me and only said what had to be said. Her large body swayed to and fro as she slowly went through all of her procedures before she went out to call the doctor.

Donna arched her back against the bed and groaned.

"I'm sorry, Juliana. I need something for the pain. My back is killing me."

"Donna, don't apologize. The baby is just locked in a posterior position and putting a lot of pressure on your back. You are strong and are doing your best," I tried to console her.

The nurse came back into the room.

"Dr. Gaynor won't come in. He says he knows nothing about your arrangement with Dr. Michaels. He's against home birth and he doesn't want to be involved."

Chills went up and down my spine. Why did Dr. Michaels say he would back up Donna and then go on vacation? Why didn't he tell his partner he was doing this? I knew Donna would need a cesarean, but what would I do now?

"Give me his phone number and I'll call him," I said.

"I don't think he'll talk with you," the nurse warned.

"Then I'll talk with him," Victor said emphatically.

She looked at him doubtfully but motioned for him to follow her to the phone.

He dialed the number. I stood next to him, powerless to help him.

"Dr. Gaynor?" he said suddenly.

"This is Victor Delaney. My wife, Donna, is here after a transfer from a home birth because she needs to have some medical intervention."

He paused.

"Yes, I know," he said.

Pause.

"I know."

Pause.

"Uh huh. But you have to understand. Dr. Michaels said he would back us up as recently as a month ago. We assumed then that he would be here. We also assumed that he discussed it with you since you are partners."

"Please, Dr. Gaynor, please come in and help us out!"

He was begging now. There was another pause.

"But you will get paid! I have insurance. I'm an employee of this county and I carry the family health plan through them."

Pause.

"Oh, thank you very much. I appreciate it."

He hung up the phone and looked at me. He looked haggard.

"He's coming in," he said. His voice was tired. "He knows he'll get the money."

His shoulders hung down. I put my arm around him as we walked through the icy tile hallways back to Donna's room. She had gotten herself back on her hands and knees and was breathing through a contraction.

"Juliana, I want out of this now," she implored.

"Dr. Gaynor is coming in," I told her. "He'll be here soon."

A half hour later Dr. Gaynor walked in the room. He didn't acknowledge me although we had met only six months before at another meeting.

He was not rough on Donna at all, he was just very methodical. He did a vaginal exam and decided immediately to do a cesarean section. He told Victor and Donna his findings and walked out.

I held Donna's hand to comfort her through another contraction and right when she was done, I put her hand in Victor's and went out to the hallway to find Dr. Gaynor. I don't know what I wanted to do or say. I just wanted to communicate with him. I just wanted to tell him that I could understand that he felt backed into a corner. Somehow I wanted to make things right even though I knew I couldn't. Let's face it, he was angry at me for doing home births and at Dr. Michaels for agreeing to back me up. And, I was angry at Dr. Michaels for not telling him of our arrangement before he left for vacation. I was also angry at Dr. Gaynor for refusing to come until he was sure he was being paid. How could he reduce Donna's travail and the birth of her baby to a mere question of money? I felt hopeless as I walked through the halls looking for him. How could any positive interaction come about with all of those combative feelings in the air?

The hallway was empty except for the nurse sitting at the nursing station. I walked up to her.

"Where did Dr. Gaynor go?" I asked. My voice seemed to echo in the quiet darkened halls.

She didn't look up from her paperwork.

"He's changing," she answered.

I waited for awhile in the halls. He didn't come out. I went back to Donna. The anesthesiologist was starting an epidural. The nurse prepped her and put in a catheter. Finally she was ready to be wheeled back.

I watched the entourage disappear behind the doors of the operating room. I turned and slowly made my way to the lobby. I was exhausted and emotionally drained.

The elevator inched down to the main floor. It seemed like it stopped between the floors. Somehow I hoped it would so I would remain there blankly suspended in time and space and not feel my feelings.

The elevator opened on the ground floor. The lobby was empty except for Victor's mother and a friend. They both looked up expectantly as I walked out. I sat down next to them on the sofa.

"They're taking her in for a section," I said.

I put my head in my hands. I was sad for Donna and Victor that the birth of their child was reduced to the level of money. I was angry at the doctors for taking their commitment so lightly and for reducing a proud and happy father to a desperate begging man. I was angry with myself for being so naive.

After I heard that Donna delivered a big healthy boy I left the hospital with a heavy heart. On my way home I stopped by Debra's house to see how her birth went. When I arrived I came upon a hustle and bustle that was not typical of a peaceful postpartum. Indeed, I let myself in the door and went back to the bedroom only to find Debra still laboring and Ann sitting by her bedside. There were many people in the room and the atmosphere was jovial.

They looked up as I entered.

"Hello! How are you? Yea! We're glad you made it," a chorus of voices sang out.

I felt good to be welcomed somewhere. I hugged Debra and plopped down on the bed beside her. I asked Ann how she was doing.

"Oh, I'm fine," she answered in her tangy English accent. "Debra just woke up from a nap and I haven't checked her yet but I think she has a long way to go. The baby is doing fine."

After a social chat Ann went to work. Debra's labor got more active. I did a vaginal exam and she was six centimeters dilated.

The day grew into a pleasant one with the sun shining and a gentle breeze blowing. The many people at Debra's house emanated a peaceful, joyful expectancy. Everyone was willing to help out. It was a relaxing, healing atmosphere from my harrowing hospital transfer a few hours before. I received a warm back rub and finally calmed down.

I spent the whole day at Debra's house. Her labor stopped and started over and over again. She progressed slowly to eight centimeters. I was baffled. This was her third baby. She should be progressing more quickly. But when I did a vaginal exam, the baby's head didn't seem to be coming down. A pocket of amniotic fluid in front of the baby's head prevented its descent. I knew the bag of waters would have to break to let the head come down, but I couldn't break the bag of waters safely with the baby's head so high because of the danger of the umbilical cord washing down in front of the baby's head and becoming compressed. I was in a bind.

I outlined my dilemma to Dan, her husband. He was a nurse and it was easy to explain things to him. He came up with a great idea.

"Let's turn Debra upside down!" he exclaimed.

I looked at him doubtfully.

"No, I mean it," he said excitedly. He was on to a grand plan.

"If we put her on her hands and knees with her hips up in the air and her chest down on the bed, the baby's head will float to the cervix and the water will drain down behind it. Then, when we turn her back over, the head will have lost the pocket of water in front of it and then be better able to come down."

I knew what he meant. Right now the baby's head was like a buoy in water. It was floating around and unable to sink. By putting Debra upside down, the water that was in front of the baby would drain back into her uterus and the head would replace it. Then I could pass a needle through the bag in a few places and let the water leak out slowly. It was worth a try.

For the next hour Debra labored on her hands and knees with her hips up in the air. Believe it or not, she actually felt more comfortable. She had been feeling a lot of pressure from the pocket of water and this position relieved her.

Finally I turned her over and checked her vaginally. Sure enough, Dan's plan worked. The pocket of water had virtually disappeared. Now I carefully passed a needle through the bag of waters at about five different places so that the amniotic fluid could leak out slowly.

The water leaked out of Debra's vagina slowly at first, making quite a puddle on the bed. It kept leaking and leaking; it seemed endless. I started scooping it into a bowl, like I was bailing water out of a sinking ship. There was a little more than the normal amount of fluid in there.

Suddenly Debra had an urge to push. I wasn't surprised. I knew that once we took all of that resistance away, her baby would be able to come down into the vagina and be born.

I changed my gloves.

The room was chaotic. Everyone rushed to their pre-assigned positions. Debra needed support while she squatted on the bed. Her father and a friend held her from the back while her husband and another friend held her sides. Her teen-age daughter hugged Debra's mother as they both watched from the door.

"A boy!" It was a big boy! Everyone was screaming with delight. His little face puckered up before he wailed with life. He was gorgeous. He weighed ten pounds and four ounces! He nursed right away and everyone scurried to prepare both mother and baby for rest. I stayed awhile to socialize and then drove home exultant, and exhausted.

The bomb dropped a few weeks later. Donna called one evening just as I was sitting down to dinner.

"Hi, Juliana. I just got back from a visit to Dr. Gaynor's office," she said. "I don't want to upset you, but I thought you ought to know. Dr. Gaynor said he was going to report you to the Board of Nursing. He accuses you of mismanaging my labor."

I sank down in the chair.

"How does he think I mismanaged it?" I asked.

"He thinks you mismanaged the second stage . . . the pushing," she answered. "I tried to tell him that you didn't, but he didn't stay around to listen to what I had to say. I'm sorry. Let me know if there's anything I can do for you."

I hung up the phone and hung on to Eric for support.

He was angry.

"The guy's practice promises to back Donna's birth up and then he refuses to come in when she needs him! Now he's accusing you of mismanagement? That's the pot calling the kettle black! I think you ought to report him!"

I thought about what he said. He was right. I knew I didn't mismanage Donna's labor. In fact, this was one labor where I kept pretty much to the textbook. I was tired. I didn't want to go through this again.

"It's harassment, Juliana," Eric persisted. "They're not going to stop till they get rid of you."

I had a sleepless night. I tossed and turned. This was another case of a doctor harassing me because he thinks he should be the only one delivering babies. More important, did he have the right to refuse care to someone because he disagreed with them about how they chose to live their lives? What if we started doing that in emergency rooms? "No ma'am, sorry, we won't treat your child here because you didn't put her seat belt on." Or, "No sir, sorry, we won't treat you for your heart attack because we think you ate too much cholesterol."

We would never consider refusing care to the majority of people who seek health care. The simple fact that a woman is refused health care because her belief differs from the doctor's is unique to the system. It reeks of discrimination against women and children.

I woke up to the bright morning with heavy eyes. I knew what I had to do. I had to treat fire with fire. I went to the typewriter to write my complaint to the Board of Medicine about this doctor's practice. I was filled with trepidation, but my sense of survival spurred me on. I didn't know if this would save me, but at least I wasn't going to go down without a fight. Soon afterwards I received a letter from the Board of Medicine saying that Dr. Gaynor was not in violation of his license. He had never followed up on his threat to report me. Besides my political troubles, the most tragic thing that ever happened to me in my life happened that summer. My mother died.

Early in the spring of 1986 my father called me. My mother was doing poorly on her medication for Parkinson's disease. She was more disoriented and her body was stiffer. It was harder for her to get around. And, when she got around, it was harder for her to stay lucid about what she was doing. I hung up the phone knowing that I must go to her.

But, how could I get away? I was committed to so many people for the spring. And, patients who choose midwifery care don't take too kindly to their midwife leaving right around their due date. I looked at my schedule through the months. April, May and June were all filled. But July looked better. I only had one person due and one person for hospital labor support. I decided I would go then.

I decided not to tell my parents yet that I was coming. I didn't want my mother to get too excited and then be disappointed if my plan went awry.

My July couples were upset. They understood my predicament, but that didn't alleviate their disappointment. The couple who wanted me for labor support quickly found someone else, but the other couple stuck to the hope that I would be able to deliver their baby before I went. They were due on July 14 and I was leaving on July 10. Ellen had had two of her previous children early so her hopes were high. To cover her bases though, we had another midwife on standby to help them out.

I'm sure it was hard for Ellen to spend the last part of her pregnancy worried about who would deliver her baby. For three nights in early July she called me with episodes of contractions, which always stopped after a few hours. Finally she called me the morning before I was to board my plane for Holland.

"I've been contracting all night," she told me. "I'd like to try the castor oil today. I think it will work."

She drank four ounces of castor oil. Castor oil is an old remedy that often encourages labor, especially if the time is right. It usually gives the woman diarrhea within two hours and then within two more hours her contractions will begin. Hopefully they continue and her labor progresses to the point of no return. Sometimes, though, they can stop and the woman just experiences a hard false labor. So, if the time isn't right, it can be awful. It's very discouraging.

It was a few hours before Ellen called me again.

"My contractions are picking up a little bit. They're every five minutes and they last about a minute," she told me. "They've been this way for about an hour."

I drove out to her home. I checked her vaginally. Her cervix was about five centimeters dilated. Because this was her third baby, I decided to stay. And I felt she needed my attention because of my impending departure.

We spent the day together. We walked, we talked. The country roads on which we walked were cool and shady even though the hot July sun was rising up in the sky. We stopped occasionally, sometimes for her to breathe through an especially hard contraction, sometimes for me to listen to the baby's heart rate, and sometimes for me to pick blackberries from the occasional succulent patch along the roadside.

We must have walked miles. She didn't want to stop. She was determined that her labor would keep on going. She wasn't going to let it stop and walking was, if nothing else, a symbol of her determination. Stopping would have meant failure to her. If her labor would stop for any reason, she would have blamed it on the fact that she stopped walking.

The day wore on. Her husband came home from work. We had dinner. They showed me around their garden. I finally talked Ellen into resting. Surely she needed to quiet down. Her uterus would need the energy that she might be taking up by continually moving. That made sense to her. She went to bed.

I called our birth assistant. She came and I went to sleep on the couch. My mind was so tired that I let it go blank. I was determined to think only in the present. I wasn't going to think in the future.

At about 2:00 A.M. my birth assistant called me to come check Ellen. Her contractions were every one to two minutes and she wanted to know how dilated she was. She was eight centimeters, only two more to go. She was laboring hard now. She breathed more purposefully and had to concentrate more on relaxing. I got her up and helped her into the bath. Maybe that would relax her.

She ended up sitting on the toilet for a long while. I sat next to her. My mind drifted as I sat on the bathroom floor, studying it.

"How many hours have I spent in people's bathrooms?" I thought to myself. I study fixtures, curtain designs, floor coverings and towels.

"I wonder what motivates people to pick the designs they pick. Why did they choose this particular color combination? Did they spend hours picking things out or did it all just come together haphazardly like in my home? Did they ever imagine while they were designing their bathroom that they would be sitting in there for hours having their baby with their midwife? Surely they didn't because otherwise they would have wall to wall carpeting, a refrigerator and a jacuzzi in there.

My mind went into its spaced-out mode—the mode your mind enters after working all day. The trouble is, I often don't come home from work like most people do, so my mind has to operate in the working mode for hours and days at a time. I have found that I've been able to operate in the working mode for excessively long periods if I allow myself short space outs throughout my day.

Suddenly my space out ended. I ran my fingers through my hair and held my head in my hands.

"What are we going to do here?" I thought to myself. "How is this going to turn out? I've got to get on that plane! It leaves at 12:00 noon. I've got to be at the airport at 10:00 A.M. That means I have to leave my house at 8:00 A.M. That means I have to leave here at 7:00 A.M. It's 4:00 A.M. now. I can't stay here much longer.

Desperation started overtaking me. I could find no way out of my predicament. I couldn't take her to the hospital to deliver. Ellen would never agree to that at this stage. She herself was a nurse and a birth assistant for many home births. She hated hospitals and avoided them at all costs during childbirth. She wanted absolutely no interventions.

I imagined what the hospital staff would do if I brought her in. "Here," I would be saying. "This patient needs to be delivered and I can't do it because I have to catch a plane in an hour."

"No, no, no," I shook myself back to reality.

I knew the dangers of becoming self-absorbed in this job. As soon as one puts the birth of a child secondary to other activities in one's life, the trouble begins. It leads one to interfere. Start the pitocin! Bring out the forceps! Polish the knives!

I leaned forward. I was going to put my full attention into this. I had no control over the future. But I had helped to create this situation and I was going to commit to it to the fullest. By God, a baby was being born! What was the matter with me anyway?

I breathed with Ellen, wiped her brow and supported her back. I encouraged her to stay in the "here and now." It was hard for her. We moved to the dark bedroom and sat in a chair. I listened to the baby's heartbeat. Suddenly something was wrong. The heartbeat had jumped up to 180 beats per minute through a contraction. Ellen was experienced enough to read the consternation on my face.

"What's wrong?" she asked when her contraction was over.

"The heartbeat was 180 through the last contraction," I told her.

"That's because it's moving around now," she answered. "It always moves around at this time of the morning."

"Let me listen through a few more," I said.

I knew that she was watching me like a hawk. She was trying to figure out how worried I was. She also was trying to assure me that everything was okay. It was hard for her to take this on while she was dealing with these contractions. I could tell she was getting upset.

Through the next contraction the baby's heart rate went up to 180 again. I kept my hand on her abdomen. The baby was moving around. That would explain the heartbeat rising because it always does when they're active. But we midwives doing home births don't like anything out of the ordinary. We like everything to stay within the bounds of normal, however narrow those boundaries might be.

"Let's have you lie down on your left side for a little while," I said to her.

"Juliana," she said with irritation. "I know this is because the baby is moving around."

"I'm sure you're right," I answered. "But in case it's not, let's see if a change of position will make it slow down."

She moved over to the bed. I did a vaginal exam. She was almost nine centimeters dilated. I checked the heartbeat and it was down to normal levels.

"Now let's see what it does during a contraction," I said.

We found out soon enough. It was steady. The baby wasn't moving around anymore. I didn't know whether it was a coincidence or whether it was a position change, but I didn't care. It was back to normal. We moved on.

An hour later she suddenly felt the urge to push. She got on her hands and knees and pushed for only a short while before a wonderful baby girl made her appearance into the world. She was healthy and beautiful and found her mother's nipple right away.

I didn't have time to sit and enjoy. I helped clean up. I wrote out the birth certificate. (I usually do this a few days later.) At 8:30 A.M. I pulled into our driveway to find Eric waiting for me with a change of clothes and my suitcases packed. (Never mind that later I found that he packed only one pair of underwear for each of us!) I jumped back into the car and he whisked me away to the airport.

I remember July of 1986 vividly. My mind still travels back through the pain and confusion of that month.

My trip to Holland was long and arduous. I had a six hour stop over in Boston. The crowded airport with its hard plastic chairs, cold tile floors and crummy fast food cafeterias made the long wait painful. My back ached. My children tried hard to make me comfortable. Finally we got on the plane and I promptly went to sleep. I woke up several hours later to find that the flight attendants had taken care of my children and even had a warm meal waiting for me.

My sister Willemien was waiting for me at the airport in Holland. My mother was in the hospital. When I had called a few weeks before to tell her I was coming, she got so excited that she got out of bed, went downstairs and promptly fell down and broke her hip.

"Daddy is waiting at home for us," Willemien said. "He's anxious to take Anneke and Ahren to the hospital right away. He's hoping that seeing them will make Mother want to get better."

I turned and looked at my children now asleep in the back seat. I knew how much she loved them. After living with us through my midwifery school, she had become enraptured with little Ahren, and he with her. They had a wonderful relationship. After she left us to go back to Holland, I had worked hard to keep that relationship alive by talking to Ahren about my mother whenever the opportunity arose. We also exchanged videotapes. I didn't want Ahren to forget anything about her—her looks, her sounds and the feel of her.

We pulled up to my parents' house. My father was waiting outside the door. He didn't even want us to stop the engine. After a welcome hug he shuffled me into the back seat with the children and got in the car.

"We have to hurry. Visiting hours are only between 12:00 and 1:00. It's 12:05 now," he announced in Dutch.

Willemien sped to the hospital. We hurried after my father into the building. I was amazed at how fast he could walk. His long legs stretched easily into a massive gait. He bounded across the lobby in seconds. I struggled to keep up with him.

Soon we were in my mother's room. She was lying on the bed staring up at the ceiling. She turned her head vaguely toward the door as we opened it. My father excitedly announced our presence.

"Look who's here," he announced as he rushed to the side of the bed and kissed her. I joined him. She looked at me with her usual happiness tempered by her need not to demonstrate her emotions too strongly.

I leaned down to kiss her cheek. It felt waxy to my lips. I sensed a hopelessness, a hollowness in her. My father brushed me aside, scooping Ahren up in his arms.

"Now, here he is," he announced triumphantly, hopefully. It was as if he finally produced the key to my mother's happiness. He so desperately wanted her to become normal again, to have something to live for. He didn't want to understand that a short visit from us was not what was going to give her hope. She wanted to be with us always, not just a month.

She greeted Ahren the same way she greeted me. My father's hopes were dashed. She didn't have the energy to be ecstatic. Her soul, her innermost self, was leaving her. What was lying on the bed that day was the empty shell.

A hopeless feeling washed over me. We sat through the hour. I told her about our trip and my last delivery. Suddenly she looked at me and told me that she was afraid she was going to die. I knew then that she would. Her fall wasn't an accident. She didn't have the will to live anymore. She didn't want to struggle with this illness day in and day out just waiting for our annual visits. Whether or not she knew it, she was planning to die at this visit. She was merely waiting for us to be there with her.

The nurse told us our hour was up. I didn't want to leave. My heart screamed out as my exhausted body followed my father to the door. My brain couldn't function anymore. I had been up for two nights and jet lag was taking its toll. At home I fell into a long and deep sleep.

The following week was dotted with daily visits to my mother. As I look back, I am ashamed that I let the system in Holland prevent me from staying with my mother, from holding a vigil beside her bed, from letting her know that I was there with her. The Dutch system is very particular. They believe that the elderly and sick are overstimulated by constant visitation and the best way to handle sickness is quiet and solitude. My father was very tied up in this philosophy. Whenever I mentioned wanting to stay with her, he would quickly abolish such a consideration. It wasn't good to overstimulate her, he would mumble. I relented. I knew I could excite my mother with my controversial chatter. I could put the fire back in her eyes and the rebellion back in her heart.

My father was afraid of this. He desperately wanted her to comply with her care. It was her modus operandi to rebel, and he was afraid that at any moment she might struggle to get up, patter quietly down the hall and make her escape. He would have to live with the consequences, not me. I was leaving in a month. He would have to care for her until the end. Finally I chose to preserve my father's sanity since my mother's was gone.

The morning of July 17 dawned brightly. It was the day before my thirty-fourth birthday. In the evening we received troubling news from the hospital: My mother had developed a slight fever and they had started her on antibiotics. She was resting well, however, my father assured me, and everything was under control.

I went upstairs to take a bath. The heat was soothing, so I relaxed back into the tub. I stared at the ceiling, but soon the stark white tiles were too painful to look at so I closed my eyes and sank into a light sleep. Suddenly I was assaulted by a mind bomb.

I jumped up in the bathtub. My startle was so severe that water splashed up the steep sides of the tub and crashed on the bare tile floor. My eyes were wide open and my brain screamed.

"Tomorrow is my birthday. My mother is going to die."

I was paralyzed. "She's going to die. She's going to die. She's going to die." The thought tumbled through my brain in rhythm with the pounding of my heart.

Eventually I forced myself to lie down and let the water engulf me. My mind began to slow down. Intellectual reasoning began to take over.

"Now stop, Juliana," I said to myself. "Don't be ridiculous. She just has a slight fever and they said it was under control."

When I climbed out of the tub it was dark. I lay down with the children, but I was wide awake and my mind started up again.

"Maybe I could go to her tonight. Maybe she needs me. Surely the nurse wouldn't turn me away if I showed up. How could I get there? I could take the car. No, my father would never consent to that. He would think I was hysterical and surely try to prevent me from going there. Maybe I could ride the bike. I could sneak out and ride the five miles to the hospital."

That was my last thought. I closed my eyes to plan my escape, and when I opened them the sunshine was pouring into the room. I jolted up in bed. It was morning. How could that be?

I jumped out of bed, threw on my clothes and dashed down the stairs. No one was up yet. I listened at the foot of the stairs. I heard the water running in my father's bathroom. He was shaving. I sat on the couch and waited for him to come down the stairs.

An eternity passed with each minute. Finally his footsteps fell firmly on the stairs.

He saw me immediately. His arms outstretched.

"Congratulations on your birthday," he said affectionately as he hugged me and kissed my cheeks. There was laughter in his eyes. Usually I loved this greeting from my father but today I sat stiffly.

"You have to call the hospital right now," I said. "I don't think Mother is doing well."

His face fell. His eyes flashed surprise, which immediately changed to worry. Our eyes locked. Without a word he turned to the phone and called.

"Yes," the nurse said. "She's had a bad night. Maybe you should come immediately."

I ran upstairs to Willemien. "Get dressed. We're going to Mother now."

At the hospital we almost ran to her room. She was lying on her back, breathing hard. She was laboring. I ran to her side. She was staring at the ceiling but as soon as I came her eyes focused on me. I put my arms under her head and held her close to me. Her hand was shaking so hard the bed seemed to shudder.

"Mother, we're here," I said to her. "We're here, we're here."

Her eyes locked on my face. Her breathing came in labored gasps.

"It's okay. It's okay," I kept saying.

She responded to me. "Ya," she would say between gasps.

The nurse was trying to bathe her as I held her. Her body shook uncontrollably. She was struggling. She was in her last transition of life and she was in a panic.

I watched her die. She died from the legs up. Suddenly her legs stopped shaking. They fell lifelessly as the nurse lifted them. Then her hand lay still on the bed. I realized suddenly that I hadn't seen it still for over ten years.

I continued to hold her head. She continued to stare at me as she gasped for her last breath.

"Goodbye Mother," Willemien said quietly.

It was the only sound in the room.

I stood quietly as I watched her leave me that day. It was the anniversary of my birth and now would be the anniversary of her death. But as I watched her die, I felt that the strength that left her body had entered mine. At that moment I received her final gift of inner empowerment. Her job of bringing love, peace and honor to our world now became mine.

11

MY MOTHER'S DEATH thrust me into a search for the meaning of life. I performed the motions of my trade, all the while thirsting for answers from anywhere I could find them. Because of this, 1987 became a year of learning. Despite more problems with malpractice insurance, complaints from doctors and intransigence on the part of the local department of health, the year became a foundation for the rest of my life. I learned to put politics and turf battles in their place. I learned to forgive people for their apathy. My actions were mine and if people didn't want to jump on my bandwagon, well, that was okay. But it wasn't going to stop me. Most important, I learned to see midwifery as a blessing because it allowed me to witness the miracle of birth. It was the births of these beautiful little babies that eventually healed me and unlocked the inner sense of power that my mother had worked so hard to instill in me.

I had a fun delivery at the beginning of the year. Bea was a simple woman. She was really the back-woodsy type. She came to me because they couldn't afford the doctor and she couldn't get good prenatal care at the public health department.

I loved working with Bea. Even though she had no high school diploma, she had natural intelligence and was an eager learner. The pregnancy sparked a light inside of her. Her deep West Virginia accent flavored our sessions. Sometimes she'd stop me and make me explain words to her.

"I don't understand that fancy talk," she'd scold.

When the time came for her birth, Bea was well versed in pregnancy and breast-feeding issues.

Bea went into labor on a snappy cold and clear day in early January following a biting blizzard that left four feet of snow on the ground. She lived high up on a mountain isolated from the world by distance and lack of telephone, so we had arranged to deliver her baby at my home. Because we had that arrangement, I never did a prenatal home visit.

It all started when the phone rang late in the morning.

"'R you the midwife?" a gruff voice demanded as I answered.

"Yes I am," I said hesitantly.

"Well, Bea's in labor and havin' hard pains an' you better get here quick," the man exclaimed.

"Where is she?" I asked.

It was too late. A dial tone answered my question.

A flood of panic washed over me. She was supposed to be here for her delivery and there was no way I could call her because she didn't have a phone.

I called the fire department and rescue squad to see if they might know where Bea lived. No one did and her address was a post office box. I was in a quandary. How could I find her?

"I can't believe this is happening," I groaned as I fell onto the couch.

All I could do was wait for the next call, whenever it might be. I promised myself that in the future I would always get a map to my clients' homes.

Finally the call came. It was the same voice.

"This the midwife?" he asked again.

"Yes," I said into the phone. "And, don't hang up until I finish talking, okay?"

"Yes ma'am," he answered.

"Now," I started. Suddenly, after all this time, I didn't know where to begin.

"What is Bea doing?" I asked.

"Why, she's havin' a baby, ma'am," he said.

"I mean, how far apart are her pains?" I was exasperated with the situation.

"Oh, they's comin' pretty close together," he informed me.

"Who are you?" I asked.

"Oh, I'm Don's brother," he said. "They sent me down here to call ya 'cause he don't want to leave her for a second."

"Well, why aren't they coming here?"

"It's too late for that," he answered. "You better get here fast!"

I decided not to talk anymore and get to her house.

"I don't know the way to Bea's house," I sighed into the phone. "You're going to have to give me directions."

"That'll be hard, ma'am," the man informed me. "I jes' know how to get there m'self. I don't think I could tell someone else to do it."

"I tell you what," I said. "There's a general store at the foot of that mountain, isn't there?"

"Yes, ma'am, that's where I am now," he said.

"You stay right there," I instructed. "I'll meet you there in twenty minutes and follow you up to their house."

"Yes, ma'am!"

I drove to the store quickly. The sun was bright and the glare of the white snow was blinding. I groped in my purse for my sunglasses while I tried to stay on the single lane the snow had created on the highway. The way the sludge was splashing, I knew it would melt soon.

When I arrived at the store I saw a man in a jeep. It was Bea's brother-in-law. I drove up to the car and waved. He started to get out, but I motioned for him to stay in the car so he could lead me.

His jeep began barreling up the mountain with me close behind. Little did I know how much this guy liked to joy ride. The mountain road was narrow, made more so by the melting snow banks on the sides. The road had a sequence of hairpin turns, which my guide obviously found exciting.

At first I thought I was imagining it, but after the first few curves, I realized that he had a special technique for hitting the edge of the sludge just so that it would splash the highest. Usually I admire adults who still find ways to play, but today I was finding no humor in his game. Sludge was splashing all over my windshield and I ended up driving with my head out of my window when the grime buildup on my windshield gave me no other choice. I've driven in many circumstances, but I had never driven my car hanging out of my window while maneuvering these mountainous hairpin turns. I had to duck my head a few times against oncoming splashes. Once I was horrified to see spittle flying out of his window.

"Oh, spare me," I groaned.

We finally pulled up to a mountain cabin. I jumped out of my car and ran through the first door I came to.

Bea was lying in bed.

"These are hard pains," she groaned as she saw me.

"I told you they would be," I said as I winked at her. We had that kind of relationship. It was free and easy.

I could tell by her contractions that she was in good, active labor but she still had a way to go.

"About five centimeters," I said to myself.

After helping her breathe through a few of her contractions, I examined her. Yes, five centimeters. We had enough time to get her to my house.

As we moved slowly toward my car, I noticed that my windshield was all cleaned off.

Bea's brother-in-law grinned at me sheepishly. "I didn't mean to cause you no trouble, ma'am," he said.

I smiled at him and helped Bea in the car. Soon we were on our way down the mountain with Bea's mother and husband behind us.

Bea breathed quietly beside me as I maneuvered the car down the road. We rode in silence for quite a way and pulled onto the highway.

Suddenly she turned to me.

"Julie, I'm gonna get sick!"

"Oh no, Bea," I exclaimed. "You can't do that! There's no bowl in the car and I can't stop because we're all driving single file. There's no place to pull off!"

I knew as I was speaking that it was impossible to reason with someone with intense nausea. Keeping one eye on the road, I fumbled around for something in my car that she could throw up into. Finally I found my windshield scraper mitt. It was a beautiful mitt lined with sheep's wool that I had gotten for Christmas. I handed it to her and she held it over her face.

She sat silently like that for quite some time. I watched her out of the corner of my eye wondering how I was ever going to wash out my mitt.

Finally I said, "Bea?"

"Yeah," she answered, her face buried in the mitt.

"I hate to say this," I stammered. "But, I got that scraper for Christmas, and it's so beautiful." I was embarrassed to even bring it up.

"I know." Her voice was muffled against the wool.

There was a long silence. She kept the mitt over her face.

Finally she looked up. "It's over," she announced victoriously.

I accepted the mitt back with relief.

We arrived at my home. Our procession struggled up to my front door, which Eric opened expectantly. I set Bea up in my office and we began the long wait for her baby to be born. She labored beautifully and simply. I often say that women who lead simple lives labor more simply. There's not a lot of intellectualizing superimposed on an event that's not at all intellectual.

Bea pushed for about an hour before her little boy was born. She was on her hands and knees for delivery. After the baby was born, I handed him to her through her legs, she sat back on her knees and, with our help, she dried him off, wrapped him up and brought him to her breast. A baby and mother who go through this together are hard to pull apart, and I examined the baby while he was in his mother's arms.

Bea had a hard time nursing her baby. Her nipples didn't stick out, so the baby had nothing to latch on to. Bea's baby seemed interested in nursing, so we had a lot going for us. Nevertheless, it took us many hours of work to succeed. Even though the baby was born in the early evening, it was 3:00 A.M. before I dropped wearily into bed. Bea and her family stayed until late morning before going back to their mountain cabin.

Early in the year, politics loomed again. While I was at a Perinatal Services Advisory Board meeting I heard about the Statewide Council on Infant Mortality. This Council was created by the General Assembly to study ways to decrease infant mortality in Virginia. The Council would be made up of prominent department heads in the state, representatives from the clergy, prominent business leaders in the state, professionals involved in maternal and child health, some physicians and finally some citizen members.

I decided to try to get on the Council as a representative of a profession involved in maternal and child health. I called Juli Culver, a nurse practitioner with many political connections in Richmond, for advice. She was always helpful.

"This is a political appointment from the Governor, Juliana," she explained. "You've got to get as many recommendations as you can, but most importantly, you've got to get a recommendation from a Democratic delegate. Bill Jones, your delegate, is a Democrat. Go meet him. Meanwhile, I'll write you a recommendation myself. Good luck! This council would be great for you to get on!"

I called Bill Jones' office, made an appointment and settled down to ask various chairmen of my schools, the president of the American College of Nurse-Midwives, and my back-up physicians for recommendations. All of them gladly complied.

I went for my appointment with Bill Jones. I was nervous. I had never done anything like this before.

This man was definitely a politician. His office was stately. When his aide let me in and waved me to a chair opposite Mr. Jones, I immediately started my relaxation techniques to get a hold of myself.

Mr. Jones was on the phone and acknowledged my entrance with a wave of his hand. His conversation gave me time to look him over. He was short and stocky, his clothes crisp, his graying hair manicured. His Virginia accent was slow and articulate. Its tone told me that the deal he was in the process of making was going his way.

I looked around the room. The furniture was "massive traditional." The walls held various official looking plaques and autographed pictures of important politicians. Finally he turned to me and asked in a quiet, tolerant voice, "What can I do for you?"

"I'm Juliana Fehr, the nurse-midwife who works here in Winchester," I began.

"I know who you are," he answered. There was an almost imperceptible tone of hurry. I caught his mood and quickly stated my business.

Putting a copy of the resolution creating the Statewide Council on Infant Mortality in front of him, I said, "I would like to get a recommendation from you to put me on this Council."

He leaned back in his chair. "What qualifies you to sit on the Council?"

I was prepared for this. I rattled off my credentials.

"What makes you a better choice than one of the local obstetricians?" He knew how to ask the right questions.

My answer came almost automatically. "Certified nurse-midwives have been instrumental in efforts to decrease infant mortality rates."

I put my resume and a pile of literature about certified nurse-midwives on his desk, including the statement by the U.S. Institute of Medicine stating that we were the providers of choice for women who were high-risk as a result of low socioeconomic levels.

After glancing over the papers he looked at me squarely. "Do you have any publications?"

I told him of my two articles. That sealed it. He called his aide.

"Len, get me Joan on the phone."

In a matter of minutes he was talking to the Secretary of Health and Human Services. The conversation was familiar and slightly flirtatious.

"Where have you been hiding yourself? You're not trying to avoid me, are you?" He chuckled into the phone and winked at me.

He got down to business quickly.

"I've got a nurse-midwife here in my office. Her name's Juliana Fehr. She wants to get on the new Statewide Council on Infant Mortality. D'you think you can arrange that?"

Pause.

"Oh, you've already read her application material?"

Pause.

"Alright then, I'll tell her."

He hung up the phone and stood up to shake my hand.

"It looks like you're in."

I stood up. "Thank you very much."

His other hand was on the door, signaling me to leave.

"No problem, no problem," he insisted. "I'm glad to be of help."

As I left his office I glanced back to see him already on the phone again, leaning back in his chair, his aide rushing in with messages.

"That was easy," I thought to myself.

I received my letter from the Governor and a plaque announcing my appointment. I had to take an oath before a Clerk of the Commonwealth. With all of that done, I waited for our first meeting, which was to be in the middle of July. It was to start with a luncheon with the Governor. I was excited!

In the midst of all of this political maneuvering, my births kept on going. In the spring, my deliveries brought me many tribulations as well as joy and happiness.

First of all, two of my babies were hospitalized. The first was the biggest baby I had ever delivered. It was a little boy, weighing 10 pounds, 14 ounces. The delivery went very well. The mother's perineum had only a slight tear and the baby nursed well.

On the morning of the third day, they took the baby in to see the doctor as I always require. The doctor didn't know me, nor was he familiar with home birth. The baby had lost a little bit of weight, which is normal for newborns, but his temperature was 101°F. This can happen with big babies before the mother's milk comes in. They get dehydrated and if they get feverish, I advise giving them some water to get the fever to come down.

But the pediatrician hospitalized the baby immediately. He put him on IV antibiotics and kept him for four days. Before the antibiotics were started, cultures were done on the baby. They took cultures from his eyes, his blood, his urine, and his spinal fluid. It was ludicrous to see this normal newborn in the hospital with many sick children, including some with spinal meningitis. After much anguish on the part of his parents, the doctor concluded that the baby probably had a slight conjunctivitis and released him.

The second baby that was hospitalized was a little girl born at home to a single mom. On day three, her pediatrician decided that the baby's jaundice level was too high and hospitalized her so that she could be treated with the bilirubin lights. The pediatrician, I knew, was against midwives and home births. I told the mother that during her pregnancy, but he was the pediatrician she had used when her teenager was a baby so she wanted to stick with him.

The days of hospitalization went by. They stopped all breast-feeding. The jaundice count wouldn't go down. I sat with the mom while she tearfully used the electric breast pump to keep her milk supply up. The pediatrician continued to be antagonistic. When he saw the metal clamp that I use to clamp the baby's umbilical cord, he said, "What's this, a hairpin?"

One night the mother called me in desperation.

"They're going to take her to Charlottesville tomorrow for a blood transfusion," she wailed. "Her bilirubin count just isn't going down! It's still at 19! What do you think is wrong?"

I didn't have any satisfying answers for her. I tried to soothe her and give her confidence.

"I really don't understand all of this," I admitted to her. "She honestly doesn't look that yellow to me."

As a matter of fact, I was slightly concerned about my assessment skills. Usually I could tell when a baby had a high bilirubin level just by looking at how yellow their skin was, but this baby didn't look yellow.

She called me early in the morning.

"Juliana," she exclaimed excitedly. Her voice had a far different tone than the night before. "Her bilirubin count is down to 11! They discovered that the machine was broken last night. This morning they tested her on another machine. We're going home!"

I was thrilled to hear the news and echoed her excitement, but actually I was disgusted. All of that intervention—the constant bilirubin lights, the three-day hospitalization, the interruption of her breast-feeding and the possible blood transfusion—was due to a broken machine?

Summer was starting and I had two more deliveries before my luncheon with the Governor. At least, I hoped they would be done before the luncheon. I really wanted to go to this event and was worried that I might have a delivery the same day. However, fate was on my side and both women delivered before the luncheon date.

The first delivery was the fourth child to a family with all young children. Her delivery was long and hard for her fourth, but she did well and the baby was born right after midnight. Right before the birth of the baby, the other woman's boyfriend called Eric to say that she had started her labor.

Eric called me.

"Dave called to say that Maury was having hard contractions that were close together."

"How far apart are they? How long are they? Did her bag of waters break?" I drilled him.

"I tried to ask him all of that but he hung up right away."

"Oh God," I cried into the phone. "She doesn't have a phone! She doesn't even have a contact close by!" I couldn't believe this was happening to me again. (From then on I required a written plan from people who had no phones on how they were going to contact me.)

I went back to my client and finished her delivery. Everything went well, but I couldn't get Maury out of my mind. In fact, I was beginning to panic.

"What if she's in hard labor now and Dave couldn't leave her to go to a phone?" I thought. They lived in a mobile home in an isolated area.

I decided that I needed to drive out to her home. After I was sure my client and her baby were fine, I started out in the starry darkness to Maury's home.

The drive took an hour and a half. I tried to calm my anxiety. As soon as I found myself stepping harder on the gas peddle, I would stop myself by lifting my foot lightly, leaning my head back on the head rest and relaxing my neck.

"Calm down," I kept telling myself. "Calm down."

The road was winding. I swerved to miss hitting a group of deer that ran in front of the car. They ran into the woods, their white tails reflecting my headlights. I barely missed a fox a few minutes later.

Finally I pulled into their little road and up into their driveway. The house was dark and the car was parked in the driveway. My heart sank. It didn't look like anything was going on.

I knocked on the door and after no response I let myself in. There wasn't a sound in the darkness. I couldn't believe it. They must be asleep. After anxiously racing to their home, I found them asleep. In all of my haste, I never thought of the possibility that she could have been in false labor. Another lesson learned.

I stumbled through the little trailer to their bedroom. The small one-bedroom mobile home was in terrible shape. The insulation was hanging down from the low ceilings. The trailer was too small for this family of four-soon-to-be-five, so there was hardly any space to walk save a narrow path between the toys, tools and furniture. Even though Maury was exceptionally neat and tidy, their house looked more like a storage closet than anything else.

I made it to the bedroom. The room was a bedroom in every sense of the word. It couldn't have been larger than 20 square feet and it was filled with beds.

Maury jumped up as I entered the room. The others didn't stir.

"Hi! What are you doing here?" she exclaimed.

"Dave called Eric and said you were in hard labor," I answered. I tried not to let my exasperation show. "He hung up before Eric could get any more information out of him."

She laughed. "Count on Dave to do something like that."

She went to the bathroom. They had no plumbing so I heard the sounds of her dealing with the chamber pot. Life is hard with no running water. I heard her grunt as she got up from the pot. She really was very resourceful. She had arranged with her neighbors to use their water for her labor by running a long garden hose from their home to hers. That would save her from having to haul water from the pump in the yard.

They did have electricity, so while she was in the bathroom I studied the shadowy figures on the bed with the help of the light streaming under the bathroom door.

Dave and Maury's two sons, one from Maury's previous marriage, were sleeping peacefully.

Dave was an odd sort of man, thin and slight. He was a Vietnam veteran and had suffered severe psychological effects from the war. He held a variety of odd jobs and was never able to stick with any of them. He was a suspicious sort, with emotional scars from years of neglect and abuse as a child. I had won his trust by treating him respectfully. He told me that one of the only good things about Maury's pregnancy was that they would see me again.

My gaze turned to William, their three-year-old son whom I had delivered. His thick golden locks of hair were the only thing I could make out peeping out from under the blanket. I had delivered him in an old farmhouse where there also was no running water or plumbing, but somehow they seemed to have more hope then. Maybe it was because they were more in love then. Or maybe the scenery was more beautiful with the rolling hills of the surrounding countryside. I don't know what it was, but life was harder for this family. They were getting poorer and poorer. They were torn apart by memories of war, unemployment and custody battles that they were losing to Maury's ex-husband. I knew this new little baby would be just another mouth to feed.

Maury lumbered heavily out of the bathroom. She eased her body quietly onto the bed that she shared with her sons. I quickly checked her. Finding no problems, I decided to take a nap on their couch before heading home. I didn't want to travel on back country roads by myself with no sleep if I didn't have to.

I tried to make myself comfortable on a shabby two-seat couch in the living room. I found an old quilt for a pillow and another for a cover. My eyes got used to the dark and I stared at the shadows of the insulation drooping menacingly from the ceiling. The quiet of the country pervaded the trailer. I tried to quiet my mind. Suddenly a chill went up and down my spine. A dreadful sound filled the room. There was something gnawing on the wood frame of the couch.

My body froze with fear. A mouse! A rat! The noise was getting louder and louder. I was afraid to move. What was I going to do? My bravery as a nurse-midwife far surpassed my bravery when it came to rodents.

Suddenly my beeper went off. Loud shrill beeps penetrated the night. I jumped up, forgetting the rodents. What was I going to do now? There was no phone.

Maury came out to the living room. "You can go to the neighbors," she instructed. "They're right across the yard. Follow the path of the garden hose and you'll go to the right trailer.

I stepped out into the moonlight and ran around to the side of the trailer where the garden hose was coming out of her window. I followed it to another trailer and knocked on the door. There was no answer. I knocked again. No luck. I looked around and saw the shadowy silhouettes of two other trailers in the distance. A dog started barking. Should I chance it and go to these trailers? What if they mistook me for a prowler and came after me with a gun? What if their dogs were loose and attacked me?

The minutes were flying by as I stood beside the silent trailer. My heart was still racing. Who was trying to reach me? What was I going to do? I decided to be daring. Instead of knocking on the front door of the trailer again, I went around the back and knocked on the bedroom window. It took a few sharp raps before I finally detected someone fumbling with the curtains. For all I knew, I would momentarily be staring down the barrel of a gun. I held my breath until a head peeped through the curtains.

It was Maury's friend. I quickly explained my circumstances and she let me use her phone. I called Eric.

"It's the nurse at your last birth," he told me. "She wants to know if it's okay to catheterize your patient because she hasn't urinated yet."

"Are you serious?" I breathed into the phone. "Can't she make a decision like that herself? I told her that if she was unable to get her to urinate to go ahead and catheterize."

"I'm just relaying the message," he answered. "Do you want me to call her?"

"Give me the number," I said with exasperation.

I called her and OK'd the catheterization.

I thanked my sleepy hostess and stumbled back to Maury's house. She was sitting on the couch with an Angora rabbit in her lap.

The rabbit startled as I burst in. She held him close to her.

"Is everything okay?" she asked.

I nodded wearily.

"This is Samson." She proudly held up the rabbit. "He got loose and I found him under the couch here. We're keeping him in here so we can get all of his fur. We can sell it for $8 an ounce."

I smiled at her. I couldn't help but marvel at her spirit. She was no quitter. But tonight her labor wasn't going to start, so I decided to drive home. The dawn would break in only a couple of hours.

It was two more days before Maury called me again.

"Juliana," she sobbed into the phone. "I've had contractions off and on for two days and it's so hot. I can't take it anymore!"

I could imagine how she felt. The temperature was hitting 100°F. Her trailer must have been an oven.

"I want to try some castor oil," she pleaded.

She was a few days past her due date and she had delivered all of her other babies about this time.

I sighed into the phone. "Just give it one more day, Maury," I advised. "Maybe you'll go into labor today or tonight. If you don't, you can start the castor oil in the morning as long as you don't have any danger signs."

"Oh, thanks," she exclaimed happily. "I'll go down and get it this afternoon!"

I hung up the phone with trepidation. I disliked stimulating labor. Although castor oil was an age old method of labor stimulation, I fundamentally believed that labors should be left to start on their own accord as long as everything was normal.

The next day was the day before the Governor's luncheon. I got Maury's call early in the morning. She was about to take the castor oil. I decided to go out there right away to help her out. I knew she had the two boys and Dave would be at work today. He worked nearby, so one of the neighbors would get him if necessary.

She had just finished the castor oil when I arrived. Because contractions usually start within two hours of taking the castor oil, I knew our wait wouldn't be too long. We spent the morning taking care of the children and cleaning house. What work it is cleaning house with no running water. Luckily, she had spent the previous day at the laundromat so we only had to fold the piles of clean clothes. The day proved to be a scorcher, reaching well above 100°F. We heard on the radio that it was the hottest day of the year.

Maury's contractions continued steadily throughout the day. They came faster when she walked and slower when she sat. I made her take a nap with her boys. She got up in the afternoon, and in spite of the hot day she wanted to walk.

We walked up and down the long dirt road in front of her home. I was amazed at her ability to keep going because I was perspiring heavily. She was a tough lady. She was reflective as we walked and talked to me of her troubles. Her ex-husband was wealthy and she knew that she would not win the custody battle for her son. She had nothing to offer her son except poverty, whereas his life would have more promise with his father and his new wife. Her oldest son, a teenager with severe cerebral palsy and retardation, was in an institution. She was a teenager when she had him and the birth had been a nightmare with general anesthesia and forceps. His birth is what caused her to seek an alternative for her other babies.

I pleaded with her to go home to the coolness of the fans. She was stronger than I, but she finally relented and turned in the direction of home. I was relieved to sink into the old couch and let the fan blow on me. She seemed undaunted and continued relating her life saga to me. I'm sure I was the first person who'd ever listened to her.

Her contractions were slowing. There were longer intervals between the times where she had to stop talking to breathe through one.

"Maury," I said as soon as I felt it was appropriate. "We've been concentrating so much on your past that we've forgotten about the present! We've got to concentrate on your labor and encourage your contractions to come. You need to put your mental energy into your labor now." I held her hand as I talked.

She burst into tears. I sat quietly beside her as she cried. What a burden this woman carried! She calmed down. I got her a paper towel.

"I know, Juliana. You're right."

"Let me check you and see how far dilated you are. If you're not too dilated I want you to rest. If you are, we'll do everything we can to get the labor to continue."

Dave walked in the door and I explained our plan to him.

I checked her and her cervix was eight centimeters dilated. The vaginal exam seemed to stimulate her contractions. She had two very close together.

"I want you to start rubbing your nipples," I told her. "After every contraction I want you to wait a minute and start stimulating them until the next contraction starts, then repeat the cycle. Let's try to get your contractions three minutes apart."

She followed my instructions diligently but she barely needed to. Her contractions came easily on their own. We watched and waited for nearly an hour. Suddenly she really had to work hard to stay on top of them. I sent Dave next door to call the birth assistant and I got my equipment ready.

She seemed to know the moment we were all ready.

"I have to push," she wailed.

She grabbed my hand and held it with a vise-like grip. She groaned as she gave in to that overwhelming pushing reflex. What an animalistic force this part of labor is. She immediately became purposeful. Her groans and grunts were gutteral and her eyes were closed, showing an inner concentration none of us could break.

"The baby's coming," she moaned. Her eyes flew wide open.

No matter how many times you have a baby, that sensation of a baby's head barreling through a vagina is a surprise indeed.

I saw she was right.

I looked directly in her eyes.

"Maury, I want you to pant with your contractions now to ease the baby's head out slowly."

She did as I said. The head was more visible each second. First the crown, then the forehead, eyebrows, eyes, nose and finally the mouth and chin. The baby grimaced against the new sensation of the outside air. The body slid out. A girl! She cried immediately. Dave lifted her to Maury's breast for suckling. There was celebration in the yard. The neighbors must have heard the birth cry. I sat back and watched another miracle.

I cleaned up. The only place I could wash my instruments was outside in a bucket with water from the garden hose. I would have to sterilize them when I got home. I squatted beside a bucket in the grass and started washing. I was drenched with perspiration. Maury's three-year-old son, his face and body smeared with dirt, stood next to me and urinated in the grass while he hummed to himself.

I wiped my brow with the back of my hand and watched him. I smiled at my fate. Today I was squatting in the grass washing my instruments in a bucket after delivering a baby in a home where the parents were too poor to have running water and indoor plumbing. Tomorrow I would be having lunch with the Governor.

Lunch with the Governor. How prestigious it sounded. I got up early in the morning brimming with excitement. I started for Richmond at 6:00 A.M. to arrive by 9:00. The Statewide Council on Infant Mortality was to have its first meeting in the morning before the luncheon.

I arrived at the Jefferson Hotel, where the meeting and luncheon were to take place. It was a grand place. The staircase was the same one that Rhett Butler tossed Scarlett O'Hara down in the movie, *Gone with the Wind.*

I hurried into the magnificent lobby at 8:30 A.M. sharp. I purposely arrived early because I wanted to change out of my traveling clothes into more formal attire. I quickly ducked into the ladies' lounge before anyone could see me. I certainly didn't want to meet a familiar face while wearing a shift and Birkenstocks.

Again an amazing transformation took place in the bathroom. I went in travel-weary with disheveled hair, looking like a remnant of the 1960s. I came out a sleek businesswoman with a spanking new dress suit and white pumps. My hair was simple but neat and my make-up was spotless. I was ready for the day.

I entered the banquet room. It was large and filled with cameramen preparing to film the event. Over in the corner was a group of tables arranged in a square. There were people seated around the table, early birds like myself. I walked over and took a seat behind a name plate bearing my name.

There were two women seated together across from me. I saw by their name plates that one was the Secretary of Health and Human Services and the other was her assistant. The Secretary immediately came over and introduced herself to me. She was such a polished woman. Her clothes were impeccable and her countenance was stately. I sensed intelligence in the way she held her head and the way she smiled at me. Her handshake was warm but professional. I liked her right away.

When she went back to sit in her chair, I surveyed the people who trickled into the room. Julie Culver, the nurse practitioner who had recommended me to the Council, walked in. She had taken a liking to me at some of our political meetings and waved at me excitedly as she walked in. I envied her political etiquette and resolved to learn from her.

"How was your trip from Washington last night?" I called out to her.

"It was okay," she answered. "I'm glad I decided to come home last night so I could get some rest in my own bed."

She had called me to ask if she could ride to Richmond with me since she was coming back from a conference and her plane was landing in my area. After I warned her that a delivery might prevent me from coming, she decided she wouldn't risk it.

"Did you have a delivery?" she asked.

"Yes, yesterday I delivered a nine pound girl," I laughed.

"Nine pounds! Was everything okay?" she asked.

"Yes, both mother and baby are doing fine."

Her attention was diverted by a newcomer, a delegate from eastern Virginia. They were good friends.

I went back to watching the group. The table was filling up. There was some activity at the door. A woman entered, towering over the many people around her. Her jet black hair surrounded her face imposingly. Her stride was long and self-assured. She was at the table in seconds, sure of herself amidst the many reporters. She acted as if she had been the center of activity her whole life. Of course she had! She was Lynda Bird Johnson-Robb, the daughter of Lyndon Johnson, the thirty-sixth president of the United States. She was an honorary member of our Council.

The meeting was an introductory one. We reviewed some preliminary goals of the Council. The Secretary of Health and Human Services asked for a lot of input. The suggestions from the members were stimulating and the personality of the group promised to be lively.

Finally the meeting was over and the luncheon was to begin. As we walked over to our tables, the Governor joined us. The television cameras started rolling. A man walked up to me. I recognized him as a man who was in the audience while the Council meeting was in progress. He introduced himself as the assistant director of Maternal and Child Health in the state.

"What hospital do you work in?" he asked. His Slavic accent was thick.

"I don't work in a hospital," I said. "I work in people's homes."

His eyes flew open in surprise. He was affronted.

"How could you do such a dangerous thing as deliver babies in the home?" he exclaimed.

"I screen my patients quite thoroughly," I answered, keeping my cool. I was used to such reactions. "My statistics are excellent. Besides, it would probably be more advantageous for you to look inside the hospitals if you want to find dangerous practices."

"Whatever do you mean?" he asked, even more astonished.

"I mean," I continued calmly, "the high cesarean section rate, epidural rate, and frequent use of painkilling drugs that depress the baby's respiratory efforts. Have you ever seen a baby born to a mother who received Demerol? That baby is in a lot more trouble than a baby born naturally at home with a midwife."

He was startled by my statement but realized quickly that I was right. "Yes, I am a gynecologist and we always delivered women who were heavily sedated," he murmured.

We chose our seats, he sat a few seats down from me and I found myself surrounded by women from the fields of education and social services. Julie was sitting three seats down. We ate our lunch before the Governor's speech.

I felt awkward during the lunch. I was never very good at small talk and after our introduction, my companions and I fell silent.

Suddenly I heard Julie's familiar voice ringing out.

"Juliana," she called, bending her head around the people seated between us. "I hear you delivered a baby yesterday!" Her voice was loud and clear. Her smile hid a quick furtive glance to her companions, making sure they were listening.

"What was it, a boy or a girl?"

"A girl," I replied.

Again a quick glance around the table. "How much did she weigh?"

"Nine pounds," I answered.

"Nine pounds!" her voice exclaimed loudly. She turned to her companions. "Can you imagine?"

Turning to me she continued, "You must have had to cut a huge episiotomy for that one!"

I searched her face incredulously. She smiled at me and her eyes were bright. She was giving me an opening.

"No, she had no episiotomy," I said.

"No episiotomy!" she exclaimed with heightened vigor. "Just how did she manage to deliver her baby without an episiotomy? She must have had a huge tear!" She tossed her napkin onto the table for emphasis.

I looked at her squarely. She continued to smile at me.

"No, she didn't tear at all," I said, returning her smile.

"Can you imagine that?" she said to the people around us. "A nine pound baby with no episiotomy and no tear! We've got to learn something from those midwives!"

She jumped to another topic as smoothly as she had entered that one and left me to answer the questions that followed. I was grateful to her for adding spice to a dull lunch.

When we finished eating, the Governor spoke to us from his podium. As the television cameras rolled, he spoke to us with hope and promise. Even though Virginia had the eleventh highest infant mortality rate in the nation and many women didn't have access to prenatal care, this Council would work to change all of that. We listened attentively and clapped when we were supposed to. I was amazed at the pomp and circumstance of politics on display, but I wasn't fooled into thinking that anything significant was to come of this. Everyone in that room knew the reason for the high infant mortality rate. There was not enough prenatal care being offered. Everyone knew why. The doctors wouldn't provide it to low-income women because there wasn't enough money in it. Everyone also knew what could be done. One solution was to get more providers who were low cost yet highly effective. But these providers would be nurse-midwives and the doctors didn't want anyone on their turf. Major solutions weren't going to come about despite the glamour of that day, and everyone knew why. Because the doctors financially supported a lot of the legislators in that room.

I looked forward to delivering babies. They strengthened me and kept me focused on what was real in this world. All of them sustained me, all but one.

Darla was a secretive woman, quiet and suspicious. It's so easy for me to say that now, but then I naively overlooked my impression. She looked at her husband whenever she spoke and wouldn't willingly make eye contact with me. I guess I ignored her behavior because her husband was so friendly and jovial; he covered for her. I convinced myself that she was just shy.

Darla's pregnancy was relatively easy except that she smoked. The first few visits I worked hard to get her to quit. I explained to her my rationale for not delivering babies at home to mothers who smoked. There was a greater incidence of fetal distress with these babies, and I wasn't going to walk into a home birth with a known health risk. It just wasn't fair.

I finally gave her a deadline. She had to stop smoking by the twenty-eighth week of pregnancy or I would have to send her to someone who would be able to deliver her baby in the hospital. When she told me at twenty-eight weeks that she had totally quit, I had to trust her because I couldn't do otherwise. I based my service on a trust. I gave advice and I had to trust that people followed it. If they did the best they could, they could trust that I would do the best I could. I hoped that over the long hours I spent with them during their pregnancies, we would develop that trust. I had never been proven wrong until Darla.

They called me one sunny morning. Darla had contractions that were very mild and twenty minutes apart. We kept in contact throughout the day. Finally I decided to go to their home late in the evening even though the contractions were only ten minutes apart. I would sleep there and be close by in case she needed me.

When I arrived I noticed Darla was pensive, but as usual she hid behind her husband's cheerfulness. I made a note of her mood and tried to be especially gentle and respectful of her. I sensed she was suspicious. I did a vaginal exam. Her cervix was nine centimeters dilated. It would just have to dilate one more centimeter and she would be ready to push her baby out.

I was surprised that she was nine centimeters dilated. Her contractions were still ten minutes apart and they didn't seem very strong. I would have expected them to be at least three minutes apart and a lot closer. Her labor was almost over and she was behaving as if it was just beginning.

I sat and talked with them a little, while hoping to draw her out of her quiet mood. She seemed detached.

"Maybe she's just tired," I said to myself.

Darla's husband looked at me. "Why don't you go ahead and sleep for awhile? I'll get Darla to sleep and maybe her labor will pick up after she's had some rest."

I agreed with his plan and went to bed.

I awoke at 5:00 A.M. No one had called me through the night. I waited to hear a sound. Nothing. Finally I got up and went into the hall. Their bedroom door was open and Darla was standing just inside gazing out of the window.

"How are you doing?" I asked her.

"Fine," she answered.

"What's happening with your contractions?" I asked.

"They're still the same," she sighed.

"Did you get some sleep?" I asked.

"A little, but the contractions kept waking me up."

"Let me listen to the baby and check you," I said.

The baby was fine but her cervix was still nine centimeters dilated. What could be holding things up? Her contractions were still pretty mild. I tried to talk to her about my concerns.

"You've been nine centimeters dilated for about eight hours now," I began. "I know that your contractions aren't strong enough to help your labor progress and that concerns me."

"What's wrong with that?" she asked. I ignored the faint hint of irritation in her voice.

"Well, if your uterus doesn't contract hard enough to deliver your baby within a reasonable amount of time, you might be in labor so long that it will finally fatigue. If you happen to deliver after such a long labor, your uterus may not want to contract after the baby is born and then you can hemorrhage."

I tried to give such alarming information in as matter-of-fact a way as I could so I wouldn't alarm her. She didn't respond. Her husband woke up and took over.

"What can we do to encourage her contractions?" he asked.

I told them how to do nipple stimulation and went downstairs while they tried it.

They tried for about an hour before she resorted to castor oil. After she drank it, they came downstairs to use the bathroom. They stayed in the bathroom for about forty-five minutes. I couldn't figure out what was going on. I called in a few times and they assured me that everything was okay. I was getting slightly worried and suspicious. Finally I opened the door and walked in. There she was, sitting on the toilet smoking a cigarette. There were a few in the ashtray. I couldn't believe my eyes.

She looked up at me defiantly.

"Darla!" I exclaimed. "What are you doing?"

"What does it look like I'm doing?" she sneered.

"You lied to me," I accused.

"So what?" she shrugged, taking a long drag off her cigarette.

"I can't believe that you would endanger your baby by smoking when it is so dependent on you for oxygen. I also can't believe you would endanger my practice when we talked so much about smoking making you high risk and I'm not supposed to take on high risk pregnancies."

Her eyes narrowed. "You don't care about my baby. You just care about saving your own ass." She brushed past me and stomped up the stairs.

I was stunned. I stared at my birth assistant. I turned and walked out of the house. She followed me.

I walked and walked. My anger blinded me to everything. All I could do was move forward. My birth assistant struggled to keep up. Finally she grabbed my arm.

"Whoa, Juliana, slow down. You need to think about what you're going to do."

I stopped. Suddenly all of my energy left me. I sank down on the ground by the side of the gravel road.

"You're right," I moaned, my head in my hands. "But what can I do?"

"You probably ought to transfer her," she answered.

"Do you think she's going to listen to me and go? She's not going to do a thing I say. I feel like walking out on her."

"Juliana," my birth assistant said, "Darla's a hurtful woman. She's hurting the baby and everyone around her because she's been deeply hurt. You've always said that labor brings out the honesty in women. You just saw Darla's true side and you've got to deal with it, not run from it."

I knew she was right. I couldn't walk out on her. I've never done that to a woman in labor and I couldn't start now. Besides, I didn't want to dump her on Dr. Peterson. He trusted me to assess my patients adequately and only bring patients to the hospital who were in medical need. I also knew that, in Darla's case, he wouldn't get paid. They were poor and unable to keep up with their bills. I knew I had to bite the bullet, own up to my own mistake in judgment, and do the best I could.

I went back to her house. They were upstairs in the bedroom. I knocked. "Come in," she called.

She was standing beside her bed and breathing through a contraction. I quietly got my fetoscope and listened to the baby's heartbeat. Everything was okay.

"Darla," I said when she was finished, "I don't know how this situation got so out of hand, but I want you to know that my concern is for your baby's safety. I'll stay through your labor and I won't transfer you unless I see a problem with the baby. I'm sorry things had to turn out like this."

I put my arm around her and her husband tried to lighten the situation with humor. She smiled at him, and I had to take that to mean that she had calmed down.

As I stood beside her I realized that her contractions had changed. She had had three contractions since I walked back in the house. I watched her closely. Sure enough, after three minutes, another one came. Then another. Something had tipped the scales and put her into a good contraction pattern. Perhaps her adrenaline was all she needed.

I suggested she go lie down on the couch. She got on her left side and I listened to her baby's heartbeat again. I detected a slight drop in the rate at the end of the contraction. It happened again and again.

I looked at both of them.

"The baby's heartbeat is going down with the contractions. I don't feel comfortable keeping you at home. We'll transfer you in my car."

Darla said nothing but her look was menacing.

I put her lying down in the back of my station wagon with her husband sitting beside her. She cried out with her contractions. I tried to encourage her to breathe slowly and evenly through them.

"Oh, shut up, Juliana!" she screamed at me.

We pulled into the hospital parking lot and I backed up to the emergency entrance. She felt the urge to push. A nurse ran out and helped me. We checked the heartbeat and it was fine.

"Push your baby out, Darla," I said.

"Shut up!" she screamed.

I got up to her face.

"Look, Darla," I said in a very quiet but threatening voice. "You push that baby out right now or I'll send you through those doors and you'll be $3,000 poorer."

She pushed her baby out with the next push. He wailed and I put him on her chest. She and her husband were exultant and all smiles.

The placenta came out almost immediately and while I was delivering it, an obstetrician walked by in the parking lot.

"What's going on over there?" he called.

An orderly explained the situation.

"Get that midwife's name and license number," he yelled to the nurse who was helping me.

The nurse quickly got a paper and pencil and approached me apologetically. We had taken an immediate liking to one another when she raced out to help me with the delivery.

I closed the hatch of the car, shutting Darla and her family in the back and ran to my door. She was there waiting for me.

"I know you have to follow doctor's orders," I said quickly to her as I jumped in my car. "But that information is none of his business. Thanks so much for helping me."

I started the car and sped out of the parking lot.

Darla and her husband were happy as I drove them home and got them settled. I was consumed by anger and pity for this baby. As I packed up my bags and walked out of the house, her husband held up a bag of marijuana.

"I'd like you to have this as a thank you present."

I looked at him in disbelief, refused his gift and walked out. I cried all the way home.

My experience with Darla toughened me. In one day I had fought with a patient, transferred to the hospital, delivered a baby in my car and narrowly escaped an attack by a physician. It was all too much. I couldn't afford to be that vulnerable again. I learned to confront my patients if I suspected anything strange.

Yes, 1987 was a year of lessons. After managing a hemorrhage during a blizzard, I learned to react more quickly if I thought a woman was going to bleed too much. After yet another pediatrician hospitalized another one of my babies unnecessarily, I learned to use only pediatricians who knew me. And on the lighter side, after I caught five goats balancing on the hood of my car during a delivery on a farm, I learned to talk to people about controlling their animals during births.

By the time the year ended, I had become a well-seasoned, tough midwife. I demanded compliance from my clients. I worked hard to tailor my instructions to their needs so I took no excuses for failures to follow through with my advice. And I was more relaxed about the political scene. I saw the system as incompetent and merely struggling to survive. The threat was gone. No one could take away my competence, my knowledge, my compassion and my integrity as a midwife.

12

THERE'S ONLY ONE WAY to describe 1988: high gear. I was up to my
neck in politics, and my service was operating at peak capacity.

People always asked me, "What do you do if you have two women in
labor at the same time?"

First of all, I limit the number of people with due dates in the same month
to four. That decreases the chance that two people are going to go at the
same time. Second, I keep well stocked with registered nurses as birth assistants who can monitor women in labor. Luckily, one of my birth assistants
was a nurse-midwife trained in England. I used her as much as I could.

But even the best plans can be foiled in this profession. People deliver
early and late. People whose due dates are a month apart can deliver a day
apart, or even on the same day. A few back-to-back episodes of births added
to the excitement of my life. One particular episode happened in early spring.
This time I had five in one week.

It started on Sunday when I was hiking on the Appalachian trail and my
beeper went off. I hurried to a house nearby and asked if I could use their
phone. It was Joan, a black Muslim woman, who had beeped me. I waited
a little impatiently for her to tell me the details of her labor as I stood in this
stranger's living room. The woman who answered the door had been pleasant
but the man stared at me menacingly. I was starting to get a little antsy.
They had at least twenty to thirty rifles all over their living room and a bridal
photo of the two showed them both carrying rifles. I quickly finished my
conversation, thanked them and left. Later on in the evening I delivered
Joan's seventh child, a girl.

Two hours later, as I was sitting on the bed visiting with her and her entire
family, Eric called to say that another one of my patients had a broken bag
of waters. I quickly drove home to catch a few hours of sleep before traveling
to her home in the wee morning hours. She delivered her first baby, a boy,
that afternoon. I rested for a day and then held my office hours into the
evening on the next day.

The next morning I was called to another delivery. This was the first baby
for a family living in a cabin in the mountains. Rick, the father, was a

photographer and Janine, the mother, was a social worker. They were excited about their pregnancy and this upcoming delivery.

When I arrived, Janine was laboring well. I did a vaginal exam and felt an intact bag of waters. I was confused by my vaginal exam. Her cervix was six centimeters dilated but the head didn't feel like a head. It felt more like a breech presentation, but I was sure that I could feel the head when I pressed down on the outside of her abdomen.

"I'm confused about this vaginal exam, Janine," I said. "The baby's heartbeat is fine and there are no danger signs, but I can't tell if the head or the breech is down."

She was calm. "I don't think I felt the baby turn at all," she said. "Isn't the heartbeat in the right place for a head-down position?"

"Yes, it is," I answered. "I'll continue to monitor the baby and I'll check again in a half hour. It's certainly no emergency. If it is breech, we'll have enough time to get you to the hospital."

Again my findings were confusing, but I leaned more toward the breech theory. I felt a bony crease that felt similar to the suture on the baby's skull. But because there was soft fleshy tissue on either side of the crease, I was inclined to believe that it was the crack of the buttocks, even though they never felt like that to me before.

I decided to take her to the hospital. She progressed quickly and was already nine centimeters.

I put her in the back of my car on her side. My birth assistant drove and I stayed in the back with her to monitor her and the baby. Rick followed in his car.

On the way to the hospital she felt an urge to push and I checked her to find that she was ready. I encouraged her to pant with her contractions so that the pushing would be slow and gentle. By the time we got to the hospital, I could see some of the baby at the vaginal opening. It looked like lips that were presenting, but because I felt that bony crease I still held onto my breech theory and felt that they were swollen labia. Still, I encouraged her to slow down.

"Breathe evenly and try not to push," I whispered to her as we pushed her stretcher up to the delivery room.

Dr. Wemsah had been warned by my phone call before transfer, so he was on his way.

We put her on the delivery table and I delivered the baby. What I saw confirmed a fleeting consideration that I held earlier. The baby's face was coming first. But what was the bony ridge? As the face came out into my hands, I saw immediately that it had a severe cleft lip and palate.

The baby was born. She wailed right away. Dr. Wemsah walked in.

"What's the matter with her?" Rick asked in alarm.

I knew the task ahead was going to be hard. I breathed a deep breath and tried to sound as calm and forthright as possible. I remembered from my training to emphasize the positive aspects of the baby as much as possible.

"She has a cleft lip and palate," I answered.

Dr. Wemsah took over the delivery of the placenta so that I could talk to Janine and Rick.

The baby was taken over to the warmer to be dried off and suctioned. I walked over to watch her.

"She looks so healthy," I said.

Indeed she did. She was beet red and screaming. I tried to hurry the nurse up. Finally, I helped her wrap the baby up to bring her to her parents. As I did, I noticed that the two middle fingers on both hands were partially missing.

"Two separate defects are worse than just one," I thought to myself. It could mean an entire syndrome was present.

The baby looked pretty bad with the clefts and the swollen face from the delivery. Face presentations always look so awful. I knew that when the baby looked so bad, bonding can be especially difficult. All I could do was place the baby on Janine's chest. She wept as she soothed her baby's cries.

"Babies that are born face first always have swollen and bruised faces. The swelling will go down in the first few days," I started.

"Will she be able to have surgery to fix her lip?" Rick asked anxiously. Janine was still busy soothing the baby and cooing to her.

"Yes," I answered. "It's usually done over a few months because they have to do it in stages."

Janine grasped her hands and noticed her fingers.

"What's this?" she asked in alarm. This seemed to hit her harder than the lip.

"It looks like her fingers didn't develop normally," I said. "Her other hand is the same."

"Why?" Janine whispered.

Rick was quiet. I could tell he was deeply disturbed at the sight of his daughter.

"I don't know, Janine," I said. "We'll have to talk to the pediatrician."

I stayed with them for a while after the birth. They seemed to gather their strength. By the time I left, Janine was settled in bed. The pediatrician had come and they were making plans to transfer the baby to a children's hospital.

Janine went with her baby to Children's Hospital where it was decided that it was just a coincidence that the baby had two separate birth defects. They attributed the lack of growth in her fingers to amniotic fluid binding, a rare condition where she must have had her hands together in the womb and poked them through the bag. When the bag grew back around those two fingers, it cut off the circulation to them. It was a fluke. In the end, Janine's baby went through numerous surgeries to repair her cleft lip. Today she is a normal, healthy little girl.

I got home at 9:00 P.M. from Janine's delivery and at 10:30 P.M. the phone rang and I rushed to deliver another baby, a little girl, the fifth baby for a deeply religious family who lived in a cabin in the hills. I envied their simple life. Why did I make my life difficult by plunging into one of the most difficult and controversial professions in society today? Why couldn't I be satisfied with the simple things, a small rustic cabin, a few children, a garden and some animals? I knew why. Even though part of me wanted that, I couldn't isolate myself while I knew that families were going through unnecessary pain and cost in the name of routine medical procedures that created havoc. Still, as I left them peacefully in their beds, I glanced back to their home with a flash of longing.

In the spring of 1988 I went through a major life passage. I was taking a walk with the kids on a beautiful morning a week before Mother's Day. Suddenly I felt a catch in my throat, a small gag. I vaguely recognized the feeling. I knew I had it once before, but I couldn't quite remember when or why. I walked along quietly trying to figure this out.

I stopped dead in my tracks. My eyes were wide with shock. I was pregnant!

"Mom, what's wrong?" Anneke cried.

"Oh, nothing." I collected myself quickly. I wanted to sort this out alone for a moment.

"Mom, come off it," she said, rolling her eyes. "Come on, let it out."

My Anneke. My alter ego. She doesn't let the smallest bit of my life go by unnoticed.

"Okay," I confessed. "I may be pregnant."

"But Mom, you haven't missed a period yet," she insisted. (See what I mean?)

"I know," I said. "But I feel this gagging sensation that I only felt when I was pregnant with you guys."

"Mom thinks she's pregnant, Dad," Ahren announced when we walked into the house.

Eric was excited and I'd always wanted a third baby too.

But planning a pregnancy and being pregnant are two entirely different things. My pregnancy threw me into upheaval. I went through what all women go through. How could I do this to myself? Everything was going so smoothly in my family. Why would I want to make us all so vulnerable by introducing the unknown factor of a new child? I was going to be thirty-six when this baby was born. What if it was born with birth defects? We didn't have maternity insurance, nor insurance for a new baby. We only had catastrophic insurance. What if I developed complications in the pregnancy? Where would I go? What would I do?

For a while I clung to the thought that maybe I was wrong. Maybe my period would start. But by Mother's Day, all doubt was gone. The gagging sensation was almost continual. I knew it wasn't a common sign of pregnancy, but many of us have unique signs. This experience reminded me to listen to women when there seemed to be a discrepancy in their due dates. Women know these subtle changes and often have a better feel for their due dates than our sonograms.

By the beginning of June the gagging turned into nausea. In fact, my nausea was so intense that I was in bed for most of the day. I struggled through my office hours, pretending that nothing was wrong. Periodically I excused myself to go downstairs to hang over the toilet for a few moments. When I finished I brushed my hair, splashed my face with water and resumed my prenatal visits with a smile. Just about everything made me sick, especially watery things. Fruit and vegetables were out and crackers and toast were in. I even sat outside while Eric cooked because I hated all smells.

Births took an almost insurmountable amount of effort. If I stayed up all night, I'd be so nauseous I couldn't see straight. Usually I'd put my laboring women in the bathtub while I hung over the side and rubbed their backs. It felt good to hang over the cool rim of the bathtub. At one birth I fell in love with Grape Nuts and started carrying them with me.

I was reluctant to tell anyone except my family and my close friends that I was pregnant. I wanted my privacy. Because of my work I had gained a certain amount of notoriety in my area and it seemed like everywhere I went people knew me. For now my pregnancy was something I wanted to keep to myself.

My family teased me relentlessly. Every time we walked past a maternity store they would laugh and try to pull me in to look at maternity clothes. Finally, when I could no longer hide it, I let them coax me in and buy me some clothes.

A far more serious concern was my fear of birth defects. But I was in a dilemma. Both Eric and I wanted to know if my baby had any problems, but we didn't want to do anything invasive to find out. Just as I tried to avoid ultrasound and routine genetic testing professionally, I wanted to avoid it personally. But I had the same fears as all pregnant women. Birth defects are devastating, and it's hard to wait nine months before finding out if there are any.

Finally we decided to use other means of monitoring my pregnancy that were not as exact as ultrasound, chorionic villi scraping or amniocentesis, but weren't at all invasive. We would just have to live with whatever was to come.

So I started my research on my body. My first step was to take periodic pregnancy tests that measured the amount of hormone present in my blood. The amount goes up and can be used to verify a growing pregnancy. I reasoned that if the amount went up appropriately, I could assume the pregnancy was growing normally. With Eric's help, I drew my own blood and sent it into the lab. But once the level didn't go up as much as I thought it should, so I phoned Dr. Call in a panic.

"Juliana," he said. "You're working yourself up over nothing. You know those hormone ranges are so wide that they can show a great amount of variability. You're suffering from a case of knowing too much. Just relax and enjoy your pregnancy!"

I stopped doing the tests and for the next few months I took his advice. Then I thought of something else. I would do the alpha fetoprotein test on myself. That was a blood test done on the mother's blood between fifteen and nineteen weeks of pregnancy to see if there was an increased amount of this protein in the blood. If there was, it could indicate that the baby had spina bifida, or open spine. There also was a correlation between an abnormally low score and Down syndrome. Even though the correlation wasn't well researched and there was a wide margin of error, I reasoned that if I got an abnormal score, low or high, I would go ahead and get an amniocentesis.

The score came back. It was thirty-four. I knew the baby didn't have spina bifida, but I wanted to know what the risk for Down syndrome was based on that score. The lab I used didn't provide that information, so I compiled the results of a few of my clients who had used another lab and I came up with my own Down syndrome risk of 1 in 280 pregnancies. That score was appropriate for my age.

I decided to call their lab to see if I calculated correctly.

"I have a patient who had her AFP done at a different lab," I told the lab technician. "She would like to know her Down syndrome risk and I wondered if you could calculate it for me."

I gave her the needed information and heard her typing on her keyboard. I waited anxiously.

Finally she got back on the phone.

Her voice was filled with urgency. "This is serious. You need to recommend that your patient get an amniocentesis. Her risk of carrying a Down syndrome baby is one in fifty. This is abnormal for her age."

I slid out of my chair onto the floor. I felt paralyzed with panic. My heart was beating in my throat.

"How could that be?" I gasped. I tried to keep my voice normal. "When I calculated it, it was 1 in 280."

"Not with a score that low," she said.

"I can't believe it," I said. "Could you recheck your calculations?"

"Sure," she said.

Pause. The keyboard was clicking.

Suddenly she said, "Wait a minute! What did you say her score was?"

I told her.

"Oh! There's the problem! I accidentally typed in a three. I left off the four to make it thirty-four."

My hopes surged.

"Hold on," she said, her keyboard clicking.

An eternity passed.

"Her Down syndrome risk is 1 in 280. She's okay," she finally announced.

"That's what I thought! Thanks for checking."

I was still on the floor when I hung up the phone. I waited until my trembling stopped. Eric came home and found me. He reached out his hand and helped me up.

"What's the matter?" he asked in alarm.

I told him what happened.

"That's it, Juliana," he declared. "I don't want you messing around with this stuff. You're driving yourself crazy. Just take care of yourself and stay away from these tests. This baby's just fine."

How solid Eric was! I was relieved when he said this. But I never forgot how easy it is to make mistakes, even in the most astute testing situations. Had I not questioned the lab technician's first finding, I would have submitted myself to an unnecessary amniocentesis. No matter how sophisticated our technology gets, human error will always be a confounding element. We will never rise above our own human nature. I knew that as a professional, now as a mother I experienced it.

Suddenly with Eric's words, I felt a total commitment to my pregnancy. I wondered if this obsession with genetic testing contributed to a tenuous commitment to pregnancy in other women also, a commitment "with strings attached."

I settled down to life as a pregnant woman. With my nausea disappearing, I threw myself into my work with renewed vigor. I wore maternity clothes and started telling my clients I was pregnant. My baby was due January 31 and I would accept only two people with due dates in January and February. Eventually though, some friends and old clients encouraged me to take them on. I ended up doing four deliveries in January, including my own, and three in February. Luckily we developed a good back-up system in case I wouldn't be able to deliver them.

The months flew by. Because Anneke was homeschooling, I started taking her to all of my deliveries (with my clients' permission). She carried my bags for me, helped clean up, and got me anything I needed. She even helped me with a quick delivery when my birth assistant didn't make it on time.

I loved bringing Anneke with me on births. She kept me company in the car and she learned so much about pregnancy and childbirth. She got good at determining approximate delivery times by reading laboring women's emotions. Sometimes we'd arrive at someone's home and she'd secretly roll her eyes and whisper, "Boy, Mom, this is going to be a long wait!" Other times, she'd hear a certain noise a woman would make and she'd jump into action, "Come on, Mom, something's happening!"

Even Ahren started learning things about my job. He'd go with me on prenatal and postpartum home visits to carry my bags. When I'd call home from a labor he'd ask, "How many centimeters dilated is she, Mom?" That meant, "When are you coming home?"

I enjoyed doing my job while I was pregnant. I felt the baby move for the first time early one morning as I was finishing my paperwork after a delivery. I watched women labor with a different eye. Would I feel the same? Would I be able to take my own advice when it came to handling my contractions? I knew only too well how wearing labor was. Sometimes I would suddenly be gripped with panic. What if my labor was very long? I had been lucky with my last two. They were both so short. But I was older now. Again I realized that my worries were the same as everyone else's. My pregnancy gave me a valuable opportunity to develop my empathy.

Thankfully, my deliveries all went smoothly. I seemed to have long streaks where the labors were short and easy. I also didn't have any transfers.

"Boy, Mom, someone's looking out for you," Anneke exclaimed once as I lumbered heavily out to the car.

One of my long and hard labors was with a first time mother who had severe scoliosis (curvature of the spine). Doctors had told her for years that she would never be able to deliver a baby vaginally. She was determined though, and I was certainly willing to give her a trial of labor. We walked, squatted and did everything we could. Finally she delivered a whopping nine pound boy while she was on her hands and knees. She was drenched with sweat and more exhausted than she ever had been, but when she held her beautiful baby, her smile of victory was sweet.

In September, when I was about five months pregnant, I had another run of deliveries in a row. Luckily, they were all short and they never overlapped. I had four in four days.

It all started after two full days of office hours. I was called at 1:45 A.M., delivered a little boy, and was home by 7:00 A.M. Then later in the morning I was called to deliver the first son to an Episcopalian priest and his wife. They lived in the rectory, a glorious old victorian home. Church bells pealed to announce the baby's arrival to the community. We left the mother nursing her baby in their four poster bed in her white nightgown, with her beautiful dark hair flowing around her face.

Anneke breathed, "She's the most beautiful postpartum woman I have ever seen! She looked like the Madonna!"

My birth assistant, who was due in three weeks, accompanied us out to her car and slowly climbed into her own.

"See you tomorrow for another birth," she called.

"What do you mean?" I looked at her with curiosity. I thought she was referring to her own delivery. Was she telling me she was in labor?

She read my thoughts. "No, not me, you silly," she laughed. "I just meant that probably someone else will go tomorrow."

My phone rang at 12:45 A.M. It was my birth assistant.

"You're not going to believe this Juliana, but my waters broke," she reported.

"You're joking," I said. I thought she was calling to tell me another one of our patients was in labor.

"I'm serious," she said solemnly.

"You're three weeks early," I exclaimed.

"I know," she said. "Oh, Juliana, please don't make me go to the hospital because it's early!"

My mind raced. Three weeks early was borderline between a term baby and a premature one. She was determined however. She was also quite knowledgeable. She had been my birth assistant for five years. She lived close to a hospital.

"Relax," I reassured her. "Are you having any contractions?"

"They're fifteen minutes apart and real mild. The baby's heartbeat is 140."

"Try to go to sleep," I instructed. "Call me if they pick up. Monitor your temperature every two hours, drink a lot of fluids and watch for danger signs."

I went to her house later in the morning and she delivered a little boy. Everything was fine.

The next day I delivered another little boy to a woman who had a hospital birth with her other child. At that birth the doctor sewed up her episiotomy while he was waiting for the placenta to deliver and then pulled too hard on the umbilical cord to hurry up its delivery. After a beautiful natural birth, the placenta tore and the doctor put her under general anesthesia, took apart the episiotomy and scraped out the rest of the placenta. Her husband was furious with him and many unkind words passed between them. Of course, when this whole situation was over, she was anemic because of the loss of blood from the torn placenta. When I got the medical report, the obstetrician stated that she was anemic because of the husband's refusal to go along with the prescribed medical procedures. I found them to be a wonderful family, and we had a beautiful delivery that happened so quickly that Anneke helped me out.

Around that time, the local health department found a new director to replace the one who retired. The new director was a pediatrician and appeared to be a breath of fresh air. He was warm, personable and seemed genuinely interested in finding a way to provide prenatal care for all of the indigent women the doctors refused to see. He contacted me and even tried to get privileges for me to deliver indigent women at the local hospital. The hospital administrators were interested because they were forced under a new law to accept all women who entered their hospital in labor unless they were too high-risk. In those cases, the hospital had to transfer the women to a regional center. With the doctors refusing to come in to deliver these women and the cost of transfer being high, the administrators were looking for alternatives. Certified nurse-midwives were gaining a respectable reputation and the administrators of the hospital were seriously considering opening a midwifery service.

Their biggest problem was the doctors. Not only were they balking at delivering the indigent, they were also balking at allowing nurse-midwives to do the job. I couldn't imagine their line of reasoning. Refusing to give the care is one thing, but preventing others from giving it was another.

The director was unsuccessful in his attempt to get me hospital privileges. But he did convince me to come into the health department to help provide prenatal care. In the past I begged for the chance to do this. But now my service was operating at peak capacity, my political activities were demanding and it was hard to fit in another commitment. I finally consented to come one morning a week.

On the morning of my first day I arrived to find the nurses buzzing. That very morning the director had received word that the doctors would start taking care of the indigent. The health department could again start referring their patients to them, but only under the condition that the health department perform the first visit and pelvic exam because the doctors didn't want to do that.

I wondered what made them change so suddenly. Was it that the hospital gave them an ultimatum? Either they deliver those patients or the hospital would be forced to hire a nurse-midwife? Was it a coincidence that this happened on the day I started working—entering the system as a bona fide professional? I knew that as long as I stayed out doing home births, they could always present the illusion that I was the "fringe." Now that I had entered the system, I was "authentic" and I was more of a threat. My entry into the system signaled that it would only be a matter of time before my feet touched the floor of their sacred labor and delivery unit.

Dr. Way, the director, verified the news.

"Yes, I was called this morning and was notified that they would take health department patients," he explained.

"I guess there's no need for my service then," I said.

"Oh yes there is." He leaned forward. "They want us to do the initial pelvic exam and tests before we refer, and the nurses aren't allowed to do that. I would greatly appreciate it if you would stay with us and do those."

He had such a nice, friendly, outgoing manner that it was hard to turn him down. I sympathized with his predicament, so I agreed to stay.

Eric was far more critical of the situation.

"So, they got you where they want you," he declared.

"What do you mean?" I was a little irritated by his observation. I remembered the all too familiar statement by the doctors that nurse-midwives should work only in health departments with the indigent patients.

"Now they've got you working for them, doing what they consider the dirty work while they act like they're taking care of the situation. It's going to be hard to prove there's a need for your service in the hospital when everyone wants to believe they've taken care of it all. You know these doctors aren't really going to provide adequate care to these women. They're just going to see them a few times and then deliver them because they were pressured into doing that. They'd rather do that than upset their status quo by putting a nurse-midwife on staff."

I went back to Dr. Way.

"You know, I really believe that I'm not providing a necessary service here. I believe that the person who's taking the responsibility for prenatal care should do the initial pelvic exam because the information gathered from that exam could determine how the rest of the pregnancy should be handled. The doctors really should do this exam themselves."

"But they don't want to do this because the health department can perform all of the cultures for free," he explained.

"I'm sure that you all can arrange to have them send the results to your lab for free also. I do some of that in my own practice," I countered.

He threw up his hands in dismay. "I just don't want to rock the boat, Juliana. When Dr. Whitehall called me, he explicitly said that they would not do the initial pelvic exam."

He pleaded with me. "If you don't do it, I will have to and I just don't have the time. Please, Juliana. Stay with us."

Again I relented. In fact, I enjoyed what I was doing. I couldn't do a quick pelvic exam in a "wham bam thank you ma'am" attitude, but knowing the time restraints, I developed a five-minute lesson. I showed them how big their babies were. Most women had no idea of their baby's development. I compared how the baby gets nutrients with how a plant gets nutrients. I showed them a beautiful picture comparing the placenta to the plant's root system, the umbilical cord to the plant's stem and the baby to the leaves. I told them that just as it was important to water a plant, it was important to drink a lot of water for the baby. And just as a farmer makes sure his soil has good nutrients in it for his crops, a mother has to eat many good foods to make sure her baby grows well. A farmer wouldn't think of watering his plant with soda and neither should they! They seemed to like this comparison. Then I concluded with tangible advice. Eight glasses of water a day, three glasses of milk or three chunks of cheese, a meat every day and at least one fruit or vegetable.

For those mothers who smoked, I was tougher. "Would you lock your child in a garage with the car engine running? Everyone knows that's the way to kill someone. Well, your baby is locked inside of you and can't escape all that carbon monoxide you're breathing in through your cigarettes. Don't smoke! The consequences could be bad." I gave them the phone number for the American Cancer Society to get help.

For the actual pelvic exam, I tried to be as respectful as I could. I warmed the speculum before inserting it into a woman's vagina. I arranged the sheet so I could see her face and I talked to her throughout the exam. When I listened to her baby's heartbeat, I let her listen and explained why it was going so fast.

Thus I continued to provide care. Inwardly I hoped to penetrate the system the more I worked. Dr. Way was pleasant to work for, and I thought he would do anything to see patients receive better care. I was wrong.

It all started with one of my indigent clients. Her husband was out of work and they were living with friends. She was pregnant with her third baby. She went to the health department for her first prenatal visit because they couldn't afford the initial lab work.

Dr. Way found out that she didn't want to go to the doctor but rather wanted to see me. He sent one of his nurses to talk to me.

"Did you send one of your patients to us to receive her prenatal work up?" she asked.

"No," I said. "I'm aware that one patient called me for my services but she said she was coming here to get her lab work done because she couldn't afford the cost."

"Well, Dr. Way is concerned that your patients might start seeing this service as a free ticket and start coming here all the time. He wants to make sure you don't use us as a referral service. He's afraid it might upset the doctors."

"I don't actively refer my patients here, but if they're indigent, they have the same right to health department services as women seeing the doctor."

She shrugged her shoulders and we rushed on to deal with the patients.

A very short time later another patient desiring midwifery services called the health department to make an appointment to come in. This time Dr. Way called me at home.

"I'm so sorry to bother you at home Juliana, but I have a problem I have to discuss with you. Another one of your patients tried to make an appointment with us today and I wanted to tell you that the health department can't see midwifery patients unless you can guarantee that you will not transfer them to our local hospital in an emergency."

I was perplexed. "Why is that?"

"Because I'm afraid that if the doctors see in your patients' charts that we did the initial lab work, they'll get angry and refuse to see the rest of our patients."

I couldn't believe my ears. This is exactly why the system is the way it is. Everyone is afraid of offending the doctors. This fear is so strong that they're willing to look the other way while hundreds of thousands of women and babies get neglected.

"It is very rare for me to transfer a patient to the local hospital because my back-up physician works at another one, but if I have a dire emergency in this area, I might have to use that option. I can't guarantee that it would never happen."

"Well then, I cannot allow the health department to treat patients desiring the care of a midwife," he sighed.

"Dr. Way," I said, "women have a choice over who they want to see as a health care provider and we can't deny public services to them because of their choice. The indigent women of a midwifery service have the same rights as the indigent women of a doctor's service. They pay the same taxes and we have the same responsibility toward them as other citizens of our community. You're asking me to block their access to the local hospital for an emergency just because they seek my care. That would be negligent of me and downright dangerous to them."

He answered, his voice sounding slightly irritable, "When I was growing up, my family was poor and we received our care from a public clinic. We were happy with any care that we could receive and we didn't complain about not having rights. Public clinic patients don't have these rights!"

"Well, I thought I knew you to be sensitive to patients and distressed about what is happening to them in this system. If that's the way you feel, you need to call this patient yourself and tell her that she may not have access to public services because she is seeing a midwife."

"Do you understand what I'm trying to say to you?" he asked. "I can't risk losing the doctors right now."

"I understand that you are trying to do the best you can in the present situation, but we don't see eye to eye on this matter. I don't believe you can deny public services to a citizen of this community based on the decisions she makes. It's just not right."

"Okay, I will call her. Thank you very much," he said quickly and hung up.

The next day he called me and terminated my position, saying it wasn't in the best interest of the public health department to have me working for them. Meanwhile, the indigent still had to cough up $900 before delivery and then the rest after the birth to pay off the doctors and consequently were probably not getting a lot of care.

My life went on. I went on vacation and returned feeling refreshed. I had two more months to go in my pregnancy. Anneke and I did my prenatal care together, monitoring my weight, my blood pressure and the baby's growth. She read fetal development charts and kept me informed about the baby's growth and development. Both children loved feeling my belly and listening to the heartbeat. They were constantly all over me whenever I sat down. We named the baby "Yoey." Once, Anneke leaned over my belly and called inside, "Yoey, clean up your womb!" My children were my blessings.

I threw myself into my work. My deliveries were going well and my office hours were simple.

One morning in the beginning of January, Eric walked into my office while I was filing papers.

"We better get ready for this baby. It's going to be born in a week or so."

I looked at him in amazement. "I've got another month!"

"Oh no you don't. You always come early. This baby is going to be born on January 15th. Mark my words. I know I'm right!"

I scoffed at him and went on with my work.

On the evening of January 11, a client called me in early labor. Because it was snowing, I decided to sleep over at her house. At about 2:00 A.M. they woke me. Even though they were having their sixth baby, she was having a difficult time. The baby was large. Finally, after she pushed with me maneuvering the baby's shoulders, she delivered her little boy at dawn. I arrived home and commenced office hours at 10:00 A.M. and worked until 6:00 P.M. The next day was also full of office hours. On Saturday I even started at 6:30 A.M. so I could do a patient's postpartum home visit before my office hours started. I worked until 7:00 P.M.

Saturday was a difficult day. I had three new patients and because each new visit was two hours long, I had to stay crisp and clear for six hours. But this Saturday I was in a fog. Even though I didn't let on, I was struggling to keep up. I was exhausted from the past two days and one all-nighter.

It seemed an eternity before the last patient walked out the door. I collapsed on the couch and Eric pulled off my shoes. Zan came over. She had been one of my birth assistants and now she was a nurse-midwifery student.

"I was so spaced out today, and I can't seem to shake it," I complained.

"I'm not surprised," Zan scolded. "You really need to slow down. You don't follow your own advice. If you knew one of your clients was doing this, you'd be over at her house yelling at everyone to make her rest. Eric, you need to put your foot down on this lady."

"It's hard stopping her short of using physical force," he said. Looking at me more closely he added, "You seem extra out of it tonight though. Come on, you're going to bed. You're probably going to have this baby tomorrow."

"Oh, don't be ridiculous," I said. "It won't be born for at least another two weeks."

After Zan checked me, she agreed with me. Eric laughed at us. "You midwives are wrong. I know Juliana and she's delivering tomorrow."

I went to bed and snuggled with Ahren. I had three contractions in a half hour and fell into a deep sleep.

I awoke early on Sunday morning, January 15. I was well rested. I had slept twelve hours. Ahren was still in my arms, fast asleep. I kissed him awake. At seven years old he seemed still so little and sweet. He had been my baby for so long, and soon he would be a big brother. He rolled over for his usual morning back scratch.

"Let's get up. You need to take a bath and wash your hair."

I struggled out of the water bed. "Ugh, this is getting too hard," I groaned.

I started Ahren's bath and leaned over to wash his hair.

I had a contraction.

I felt so energetic. I cleaned the bathroom while Ahren took his bath. Then I started on the bedroom. Eric woke up.

"What are you doing?" he asked groggily.

"Cleaning up," I answered.

"Hmmm," he said.

I ignored him. He got up and went for an early tennis match.

I couldn't believe what a mess the bedroom was. I made the bed, folded clothes and vacuumed the floor. I had a few more contractions. Sometimes they stopped me in my tracks. Anneke came into my room.

"Mom, what on earth are you doing? You're making all sorts of racket!"

"I'm cleaning the bedroom. What does it look like I'm doing?"

I crawled in the closet to straighten the shoes. She watched me for a moment.

"Mom, are you having any contractions?" she asked. She doesn't miss a trick.

"Oh just a few here and there."

"How many here and there?" she persisted.

"Oh, about one every twenty or thirty minutes," I said. "But don't get any big ideas. I'm not in labor."

I looked around the room. "These walls are driving me crazy! Look at all of those fingerprints over there. I'm going to clean those off once and for all!"

I marched down the stairs to get the soap and water. Anneke and Ahren followed close behind. They fixed their breakfast while I scrubbed my walls.

I went to eat breakfast. As I was walking into the kitchen, I saw fingerprints all over the front of the microwave.

"I guess I may as well clean that too," I thought to myself. I started scrubbing.

"Mom," Anneke exclaimed, "what is the matter with you?"

I turned to see both children staring at me with wide eyes.

"Nothing," I answered. "This microwave is filthy!" By then I was scrubbing out the inside.

When I finished, I went upstairs to get ready to take a walk with my friend, Elaine.

She arrived as I was changing.

Anneke answered the door.

"How's your mom?" Elaine asked.

"Well, she scrubbed the walls and the microwave this morning," Anneke said meaningfully.

Elaine gasped. "Juliana, are you okay?" she called up the stairs.

"She's had some contractions too," Anneke added.

They all bounded up the stairs. They caught me leaning over the dresser breathing through a contraction.

"Juliana, you're in labor!" Elaine exclaimed.

"No I'm not! These are just slight cramps. It'll go away soon."

She looked at me doubtfully.

"I don't believe you!"

She and Anneke jumped up and down and ran down the stairs. Anneke turned on the radio and they danced around the room together.

I came downstairs. "Will you guys calm down," I said. "Look at this living room! It's a mess!"

I started cleaning up. Elaine and Anneke exchanged meaningful glances before pitching in and helping me. We cleaned the whole house and it was early afternoon before we went for our walk.

At 3:00 we went to a baby shower for me given by some community women for whom I taught prenatal classes.

My contractions virtually stopped during the shower except for one or two.

"I told you it was nothing," I whispered to Elaine.

The shower was great. The women were so sweet and I got diapers, receiving blankets, tee shirts, socks, washcloths and a baby bath. I made a mental note to start preparing my home for the baby.

"I'll start with this stuff and then build up throughout the week," I thought to myself.

As we left the shower, a huge contraction hit so hard that I struggled not to double over. I did everything I could to cover it up. I had already forbidden Elaine or Anneke to mention these contractions to anyone.

Eric was waiting for us when we got home.

Everyone was convinced I was in labor. Eric strutted around, proud that his prediction was correct. "I knew it. I wasn't going to be fooled by two midwives last night. You were wrong and I was right!"

Everyone laughed. I rolled my eyes.

"Please God, let this baby wait until at least tomorrow so I won't have to hear about this for the rest of my life," I prayed.

"You'd better call Ann and warn her," Elaine advised.

Ann was a British-trained nurse-midwife. She was going to help me with my delivery. I consented to call her, but I told her it would probably be in the next couple of days.

"All right," she said. "I'll eat dinner and be right over."

"Ann!" I exclaimed.

"See you soon," she laughed as she hung up.

I sent Eric out to get some fast food with the kids.

"Take Juliana's beeper and hurry back," Elaine called.

That was 6:10 P.M.

I called Sandy, my birth assistant. I left a message on her answering machine that I might be in early labor and to call me in two hours. That was 6:20 P.M.

A huge contraction hit me as I hung up the phone. In fact, it hardly stopped before another one started. I got on to my hands and knees for awhile. I breathed as slowly as I could, but it was difficult. The contractions never really stopped again. I wanted to run away. I made it into the bathroom to sit on the toilet.

"Beep Eric," was all I could say. I felt like I was in a whirlwind. I couldn't do anything except deal with the pain.

"I'm calling Ann," Elaine insisted.

I couldn't respond. I just sat on the toilet.

Eric came bounding up the stairs. I felt a surge of relief that he was there. I felt paralyzed. Perspiration flowed down my body. I was soaking wet. The pain was devastating. I felt like I would shoot through the ceiling or die. I didn't care which. The contractions were constant. One right after the other. There was no reprieve. There was no light at the end of the funnel of the tornado.

Eric knelt in front of me on the bathroom floor. I clutched his hands.

"Hi, honey," he said softly. His voice soothed me. I was vaguely aware of his body near me and it seemed like an oasis.

"Grab my hands and squeeze them hard," I gasped (somehow I remembered that this helped my patients so much because of vital acupressure points in their palms).

He squeezed both my hands.

"Harder," I cried.

He squeezed with all of his might.

"Boy, you're really moving," he said.

It was then that I noticed his breath.

"What on earth did you eat?" I wailed.

Another contraction hit. I closed my eyes and breathed as slowly as I possibly could as my body clamped down in a vise grip. After an eternity, it eased.

"Your breath smells awful," I cried. I kept my eyes closed. I was afraid that if I opened them I would lose it all.

"I ate some three bean salad," Eric said.

"Oh, that's absolutely disgusting," I moaned.

Another contraction. His garlic smell was overpowering.

"You've got to turn around and face the other way," I said hurriedly.

"How am I going to do that and hold both of your hands?"

Another contraction hit.

Eric figured it out himself. He ended up on the bathtub rim facing the same way I was. He twisted his body around so both hands could hold mine.

The contractions continued relentlessly. It felt like a dull knife was piercing through me while the vise was squeezing my body around it. I lost awareness of my surroundings, yet I was sensitive to the slightest change. Ann arrived.

Desperately I fought to stay afloat. Then I remembered my resolve. I remembered that I had practiced this for a long time. I rehearsed as I watched hundreds of women have their babies. Quickly I created an image of my baby behind my closed eyes. I pictured it nestling down into my pelvis. (I always told women that their pelvis was the baby's first cradle.) I pictured my baby happily waiting to be born. I pictured a glowing golden white light emanating from its body. I pictured its face in peaceful concentration, working hard to be born. The golden light grew. It spread over my whole body. I basked in its heat. It had a vibration to it and my body trembled in response. I tilted my face up and turned my palms up in Eric's hands. I surrendered myself to the force of birth. The contractions roared through me. Each made the glow brighter and brighter.

"You and I are doing this together," I said to my baby. It gave me comfort to feel I was not alone. I sent my love to my baby as it worked so hard within my body. I was happy.

Suddenly I felt something come out of me. It was the bag of waters. It was intact, just like a water balloon. I quickly got up from the toilet and walked to the birthing stool that Elaine had set up in the bedroom. The bag broke as I sat down.

The change threw me off. I cried out with the descent of the head. I could feel it barreling out of me. I pushed down following the tremendous pressure.

"No, Juliana," I thought to myself. "Stop! Pant! Don't push this baby out! Let it come on its own."

The ultimate pressure came and went. The head was out! The rest of the baby slid out and I looked down to see my baby boy in Ann's hands! I leaned down and picked him up and put him to my breast, clearing the bag of waters from his face.

He cried softly but quieted immediately as I talked to him. His eyes were wide open and quickly darted around to all the features on my face. He even turned to look at all the commotion in the room. Everyone was jumping around and screaming. Finally he settled down to nurse, his eyes gazing intently at my face.

My joy was immense. He was beautiful. He glowed with love, hope and promise. My heart poured out my gratitude at the gift I was given. I looked up at my beautiful family jumping around the room and hugging me. I realized again what a privilege it was to be a mother and to give birth to a child.

We named him Julian Hendrik van Olphen Fehr. His birth renewed my resolve to continue the fight for mothers and babies. I knew then that I would win this fight because whenever I wavered I would put the births of my children at the forefront of my cause. This was my strength because I realized again, just as I had learned from my other two births, that if I could have a baby on my own and with all my dignity, I could do anything in the world.

INDEX

About the Author

JULIANA VAN OLPHEN-FEHR is a certified nurse-midwife and coordinator of the nurse-midwifery graduate education program at Shenandoah University in Virginia.